VALUE-DRIVEN HEALTHCARE

A Medical Professional's Guide to Measuring Value and Addressing Total Cost of Care

DR. VEKO VAHAMAKI

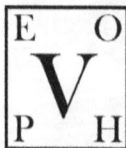

E O
V
P H

To Catalina, Adrian, and Iker—their value has no limits.

CONTENTS

ACKNOWLEDGMENTS

The endless support of my wife, Catalina, sustained the energy needed to complete this project. The encouragement of Dr. Kelly Miller provided the genesis. The clinical variation reduction pioneers Dr. Larry Shapiro, Dr. Wendi Knapp, Dr. Jimmy Hu, Dr. Laurel Trujillo, Dr. Laura Holmes, Dr. Erica Weirich, Tiffany Bailey, Ana Pagan, and Cynthia Blockinger-Lake generated the need and provided the inspiration.

A special thank you to Eric Nguyen, who proved that conceptual value could thrive in the real world.

1

INTRODUCTION

"Try not to become a man of success, but rather try
to become a man of value."—Albert Einstein

The term *value* is something that pops up almost every single day. It might be my young son forcefully exclaiming the value of his new dinosaur toy when his older brother disagrees. It might be a detailed clinical variation reduction report at work that shows decreased costs or increased quality metrics. The concept of value as an important indicator for products, processes, and services has been around for ages. Measuring value has always been a challenge, however, as both three-year-olds and graduate school–educated data analysts can attest to. Although many academics may want to favor the data analyst's numbers, there is no arguing with my son's answer when I ask him, "Is that dinosaur valuable to you?" If he says yes, then value is present. This example shows the enormous divide inherent in the complexities of actually measuring value.

Facing the challenge of mastering value measurements is akin to being asked to eat a whale. As a boy I was once faced with what appeared to be an enormously daunting school project. My grandfather wisely told me, "The only way to eat a whale is one bite at a time." That advice still rings true and should be kept in mind when reading this book, which will present more than one definition of value. Some definitions will be easier to understand than others. Calculations using these definitions of value will also vary from simple to quite complicated. As my younger son so recently demonstrated, we all must learn to walk before we can run.

Value measures can be derived from subjective sources that primarily deal with opinion and objective sources that rely heavily on facts. Some value calculations may use both types of information and will be discussed at the end of the book.

This text is designed to be a practical guide to the rather nebulous subject of value. It is intentionally presented in an order that starts with more basic concepts (Consensus Value) and concludes with advanced methodologies (combination Value Unit measures). After reading this book, you will certainly be able to understand, debate, and measure value at my son's level. Most likely you will also be able to perform some more complex mathematical feats. My hope is that both perspectives, however, will remain in your conscious as they are all part of the same whale.

2

CONSENSUS VALUE

"One man with courage is a majority."—Thomas Jefferson

Perhaps the most basic definition of value is that anything one person or several people **think is valuable,** well, **is valuable**. Consensus therefore equals value. When my young son says his dinosaur toy is valuable, is it really valuable? The answer is yes, with a "consensus" of one person. Now this may represent a slight stretch in definition as consensus does seem to imply a group. The *Merriam-Webster* dictionary defines consensus as 1: *the judgment arrived at by most of those concerned* or 2: *group solidarity in sentiment and belief.* The principle remains the same. If one person believes a product or service is valuable, then it is. That same product or service would be *more valuable*, however, if one hundred people in a group all thought it was valuable.

Definition of Value #1

Consensus Value = any subjective measure of value demonstrated by consensus measurements (i.e., any subjective measure not utilizing the Value Equation that shows a product or service is valuable to a group of people)

Now this definition has a few inherent problems. Subjective measures are by definition tainted and less reliable. In this case we are referring to data or measures that involve **personal opinion rather than facts**. *Merriam-Webster's* second definition of subjective is 2: *modified or affected by personal views, experience, or background.*

Why would we even consider measuring value from a subjective-opinion perspective if we have access to facts (objective data)?

*...because people commonly value their own opinion over any given facts. Opinion, consensus, and subjective data **can define value and give it gravity**.*

Please excuse the pun, but it is a fact that opinion and subjective data need to be measured. Using those measures to assign value is the purpose of the first half of this guide.

Take this fictitious example:
The Southern California UFO (Unidentified Flying Object) Club has 2,000 members. When surveyed, 1,800 members noted that they supported the club's provided live data stream of NASA's Curiosity Mars Rover project. (Note that a survey is a way to generate subjective data.)

The ratio of 1,800/2,000 supportive members is a subjective measure that represents important information. In this particular group of people, the NASA Curiosity Mars Rover project live data stream is clearly valuable to them. The questions to ask are as follows: *How valuable* to the group is this service? *In what way are they valuable* based on the subjective data we have available to us? The answer is expressed as Consensus Value.

Determining Consensus Value means we can look at this question from three perspectives, all staying within the realm of subjective data analysis. The first perspective involves just assigning a value score based on the percentage of people who find something to be valuable. This is called Acceptance Value and will be detailed in the next chapter. The second perspective means looking at reported use/need of a service or product and generating a Practical Value score (detailed in chapter 3). The final perspective is trying to determine if and how much the product or service creates Sentimental-Mythological Value and affects the organization that provides the product or service (detailed in chapter 4). In summary, Consensus Value can be Acceptance Value, Practical Value, Sentimental-Mythological Value, or any combination thereof.

Definition of Value #2

Consensus Value = Acceptance Value and/or Practical Value and/or Sentimental-Mythological Value

3
ACCEPTANCE VALUE

"Whenever people agree with me I always
feel I must be wrong."—Oscar Wilde

The first and most important Consensus Value measure to learn about is
Acceptance Value. This answers a key question: How much does a group of
people value a specific service or product? Do they value it a lot? Do they value
it a little? The challenge is finding a way to consistently score whether or not a
group rates a service or product in a high or low category. Determining which
categories are reasonable can also generate some debate.

Fortunately, Everett Rogers created a well-accepted premise in his 1962 book
Diffusion of Innovations. This text displayed a now-famous curve that showed
how the adoption of concepts, innovations, and belief systems follows a predictable evolution.

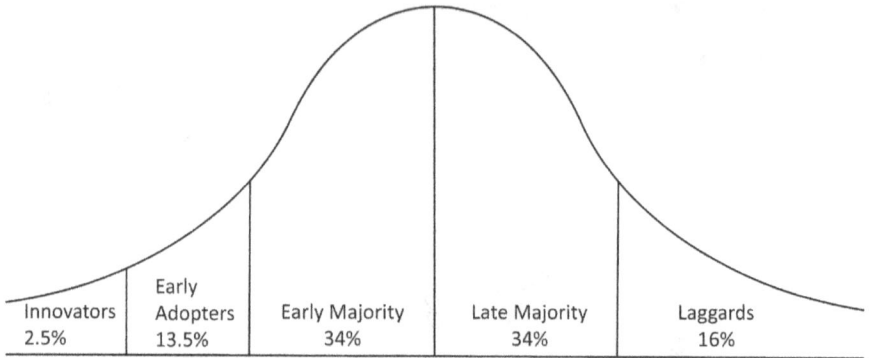

Innovators	Early Adopters	Early Majority	Late Majority	Laggards
2.5%	13.5%	34%	34%	16%

This curve illustrates how it is somewhat easy to get up to 16% of people (the innovators and early adopters) to accept or believe an idea. It is more challenging to get 50% of people (adding the early majority) to buy into the concept. It is difficult to reach a consensus of 84%, which would include the late majority. Achieving acceptance over 84% would mean winning over the most resistant "laggards."

As acceptance and adoption are synonyms, this curve conveniently allows for the creation of reproducible value categories. Since it is easier to gain acceptance of lesser percentages of people, these categories are assigned lower Acceptance Value scores. High percentages are more difficult to achieve, represent more diffuse adoption, and are assigned greater Acceptance Value scores.

Definition of Value #3

Acceptance Value = the number of people approving of (accepting) a product or service (scored as a percentage and reported as a subjective term)

Assigning a subjective score to any Consensus Value is done using the Rogers' curve as a reference. This score shows the level of subjective value generated within a group for a specific service or product.

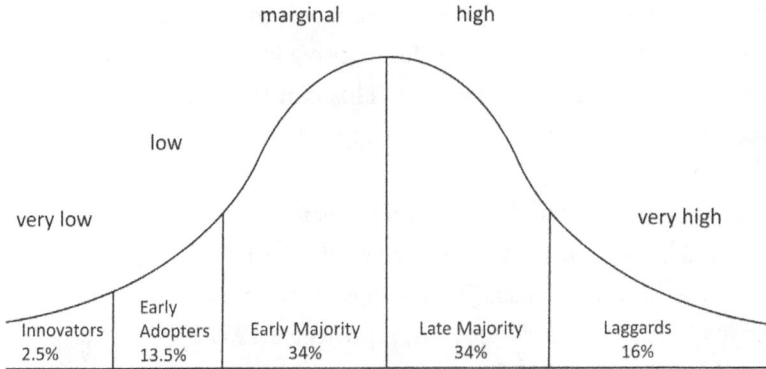

Note: Numbers are needed to assign a Consensus Value result, but the result itself is reported as a subjective term and not a number (i.e., "high Acceptance Value").

When querying for Acceptance Value, the questions should be simple and straightforward. Example questions would include these:

1) Do you think this service is good?
2) Do you like this specific service?
3) Do you give this service a thumbs up?

Let us revisit the example from chapter 1:
The Southern California UFO Club has 2,000 members. When surveyed, 1,800 members noted that they supported the club's provided live data stream of NASA's Curiosity Mars Rover project.

A basic calculation can now be made: $1{,}800/2{,}000 \times 100 = 90\%$

The subjective measure is 90% based on the survey results. As this percentage is above 84%, the cutoff on the Rogers' curve for the highest category, the Acceptance Value will be reported as "very high."

The club officers now know that the live-stream data service holds a *very high* Acceptance Value within the group. If they decide to stop this service, it will be noticed, probably unfavorably, by many people. Or will it? This data shows great support for the service, but it does not specifically determine if people are actually using the service. The club members may notice, but will they care if the service is discontinued? In order to know if people are using the service, additional data needs to be collected. This can then be used to determine a Practical Value (discussed in the next chapter).

Although Acceptance Value is a useful measure, it only demonstrates the value generated by consensus within a group. It does not distinguish the *strength or magnitude* of the consensus. This brings up an important observation about Consensus Value measurements. Just reporting an Acceptance Value (i.e., low, high, etc.) is often enough if a group does not have any subdivisions because there is *no need to compare the value.* If a subjective measure like Acceptance Value needs to be compared within a group then the size of each subgroup needs to be known because, technically, there are now multiple groups.

When measuring subjective value within a group, the n (total number of people in the group) is what helps determine which group has more value in its opinion. The n provides a measure of the strength and magnitude of the Consensus Value. When looking at the n in terms of value measures, it is directly proportional if the Acceptance Value, for example, is the same.

A group of 1,000 people can hold 10 times the strength or magnitude of subjective value as a group of 100 people if both groups have high Acceptance Value. **Put simply, the bigger the group, the more valuable its opinion.**

Let us expand on our previous example by introducing valet parking at the Southern California UFO Club:
The Star Trek committee of the club has 100 members who all support the valet parking when surveyed. The Star Wars committee of the club has 500 members who all support the valet parking when surveyed.

The Star Trek committee has *very high* Acceptance Value for this service (100%, $n = 100$).

The Star Wars committee has *very high* Acceptance Value for this service (100%, $n = 500$).

This shows that the strength or magnitude of the Acceptance Value for this service is higher in the Star Wars group by a multiple of five (500 vs. 100 on the n-value) even though the subjective score ("very high") is the same. While both groups like the service, the Star Wars opinion can be considered "stronger or more valuable" by club officers.

A few general observations about Consensus Value measures:

- A large group generates more value.
- It is harder to gain consensus in a larger group.
- A large group has a more stable consensus.

- A small group generates less value.
- It is easier to gain consensus in a smaller group.
- A small group has a less stable consensus.

Introduction to Advanced Concepts (Subjective Measures)

The only time Consensus Value measures like Acceptance Value can get tricky is when two *different size groups* who have *different subjective scores* are being compared. It is important to remember that this situation can be avoided by simply focusing on one group at a time or by only comparing groups that have the same subjective score. This should be done whenever possible as more complicated calculations are more difficult to explain to decision makers.

In order to solve this form of multivariable problem, let me introduce the concept of Value Units. The most simplistic description of Value Units would call them "points" assigned to any value measure that allows math to be performed in an easier way. Sometimes Value Units need to be created in order to have a universal unit, without which any math cannot even be attempted. This important concept will be discussed further in chapter 9.

To continue our example of valet parking at the Southern California UFO Club: The Quantum Leap committee of the club has 300 members. Of the 300 members, 100 support valet parking.

The Quantum Leap committee has *marginal* Acceptance Value (33%, $n = 300$) for the valet parking service.

With this new information, the club officers want to compare all three surveyed committees to determine how accepted this service really is considered. If this was the only group using the service, the club officers might consider discontinuing it as it only has marginal Acceptance Value. Since we cannot do math with words, the subjective scores of *marginal* and *very high* need to be converted to Value Units.

As the subjective scores represent categories rather than the raw percentages that make up each category, it makes sense to define the Value Unit based on the Rogers' curve. Since there are five possible subjective scores (very low, low, marginal, high, and very high), the five corresponding ranges on the Rogers' curve can be assigned Value Units. This Value Unit is then multiplied by the number of people in the group "n-value" to generate a result that can be compared between groups.

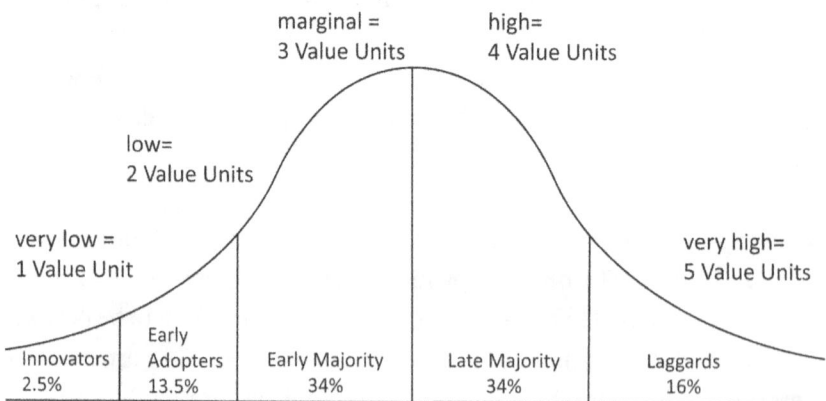

marginal =
3 Value Units

high=
4 Value Units

low=
2 Value Units

very low =
1 Value Unit

very high=
5 Value Units

Innovators 2.5%	Early Adopters 13.5%	Early Majority 34%	Late Majority 34%	Laggards 16%

Back to our example of valet parking at the Southern California UFO Club:
The Star Trek committee has *very high* Acceptance Value for this service
(100%, $n = 100$).
The Star Wars committee has *very high* Acceptance Value for this service
(100%, $n = 500$).
The Quantum Leap committee has *marginal* Acceptance Value (33%, $n = 300$).

A "total" Acceptance Value score can now be calculated:
The Star Trek committee: 5 Value Units × 100 members = 500
The Start Wars committee: 5 Value Units × 500 members = 2,500
The Quantum Leap committee: 3 Value Units × 100 members = 300

Definition of Value #4

Total Acceptance Value = multiple
of a subjective Acceptance Value
(in Value Units) and the number of
people supportive of (accepting) a
product or service

Total Acceptance Value represents a *Consensus Value and a strength-magnitude
measure* with a universal unit, allowing for many computations and comparisons to be made. A simple comparison at this point shows that the Star Wars
committee's Total Acceptance Value is so high the club officers may not even
need to look at additional analysis.

For the sake of completion, two additional concepts will be presented. Adding the
Total Acceptance Values together results in a Combined Total Acceptance Value.

500 + 2,500 + 300 = 3,300

For this combined group of 700 members ($n = 700$), the most favorable score they could achieve is 700×5 Value Units $= 3{,}500$. This would represent the highest Combined Total Acceptance Value possible for a group of 700.

Definition of Value #5

Combined Total Acceptance Value
= sum of all Total Acceptance
Values being compared

The measured Combined Total Acceptance Value can then be compared to the *maximum possible* Combined Total Acceptance Value to determine a group's Collective Acceptance Value:

$3{,}300/3{,}500 \times 100 = 94\%$

Definition of Value #6

Collective Acceptance Value =
Combined Total Acceptance Value
over maximum Combined Total
Acceptance Value × 100

The Collective Acceptance Value, representing a compiled result from both variable Acceptance Values and strength-magnitude scores, can now simply be held up to the Rogers' curve for final interpretation. As 94% is well over the threshold for the highest category (at 84%), the combined value these three subgroups hold for the valet parking service is *very high*.

The club officers now know that while the Quantum Leap committee only gives the valet parking service *marginal* Acceptance Value, the combined group of all three committees overall shows *very high* Acceptance Value for this service. It would be a mistake to discontinue the valet parking service just because the Quantum Leap committee has marginal Acceptance Value.

Challenge Problem
Now it is your turn. Consider if the UFO club survey had produced the following results. What would you do?

The Star Trek committee has 100 members. The survey shows that 10 of the 100 members feel that the valet service is good or necessary.
The Star Wars committee has 500 members. The survey shows that 450 of the 500 members feel that the valet service is good or necessary.
The Stargate committee has 300 members. The survey shows that 45 of the 300 members feel that the valet service is good or necessary.

Should the club officers consider discontinuing this service?

Answer
First determine the subjective Acceptance Value (and corresponding percentages) for each subgroup and display the *n*-value:
The Star Trek committee has *low* Acceptance Value for this service (10%, $n = 100$).
The Star Wars committee has *very high* Acceptance Value for this service (90%, $n = 500$).
The Stargate committee has *low* Acceptance Value (15%, $n = 300$).

Next, calculate the Total Acceptance Value for each group by assigning Value Units for each subjective score category (very high = 5, high = 4, marginal = 3, low = 2, very low = 1) and multiplying by the *n*-value:
The Star Trek committee: $2 \times 100 = 200$

The Star Wars committee: $5 \times 500 = 2,500$
The Stargate committee: $2 \times 300 = 600$

Finally, determine the Collective Acceptance Value by dividing the Combined Total Acceptance Value by the maximum Combined Total Acceptance Value:

$200 + 2,500 + 600 = 3,300$ (Combined Total Acceptance Value)

$3,300/4,500 \times 100 = 73\%$ (Collective Acceptance Value)

Referring to the Rogers' curve, this would fall into the subjective Acceptance Value category of "high."

Even though both the Star Trek and Stargate committees have low Acceptance Value for this service, the very high Acceptance Value of the Star Wars committee coupled with its higher member count results in a service that is overall highly valued by the collective group.

4
PRACTICAL VALUE

"The study and knowledge of the universe would be lame and defective were no practical results to follow."—Marcus Tullius Cicero

After Acceptance Value (how much people value a specific service or product) is determined, a common second component of Consensus Value that needs to be measured is Practical Value. Looking to *Merriam-Webster* again, we see that *practical* is defined as *a: of, relating to, or manifested in practice or action: not theoretical or ideal.* The goal is to answer the question: How much is a service/product needed or utilized? If something is not needed or utilized, it does not have much Practical Value.

Definition of Value #7

Practical Value = the number of people that need or use a product or service (scored as a percentage and reported as a subjective term)

As discussed in chapter 3, the Rogers' curve serves as the template for subjective scores. Practical Value assessment is no different. Only the questions used to generate subjective data are different.

When querying for Practical Value, the questions should be simple and straightforward. Example questions would include these:

1) Do you use this service?
2) Do you need this service?
3) Is this product regularly put into action or practice at your home or work?

While Practical Value scores are rarely used alone to make subjective data decisions, they are commonly used with Acceptance Value scores to further understand the value of a given product or service.

Let us revisit our example of valet parking (note that we need more subjective data to determine a Practical Value—i.e., new questions):

When the entire Southern California UFO club was surveyed again, 1,600 of the 2,000 members felt the valet parking service was good and should continue. When asked who needed or used the service, the result was 900.

Some basic calculations show the following:

1,600/2,000 × 100 = 80% (*high* Acceptance Value, $n = 2,000$)
900/2,000 × 100 = 45% (*marginal* Practical Value, $n = 2,000$)

The club officers can look at these basic results and see that the club as a whole has *high* Acceptance Value for the valet parking service but only *marginal* Practical Value. That means that people like the service, but not as many people use the service. This poses a new problem: How do we consistently explain what these two Consensus Value results mean side by side and say it in a less verbose manner? Rather than using value-statistics language such as "high Acceptance

Value" and "marginal Practical Value," a less intimidating verbiage is recommended. As will be formally presented later, all thorough subjective data sets should contain at least Acceptance Value and Practical Value components. They are the peas and carrots of Consensus Value measures and should always be together if at all possible. For Acceptance Value and Practical Value, the Rogers' curve can again be used to create a consistent language (as both these measures reflect on the individual members of a group). In the next chapter, we will see that this is not the case for Sentimental-Mythological Value.

Using standard language in place of value-statistics language when reporting Acceptance Value and Practical Value results continues a familiar, consistent pattern:

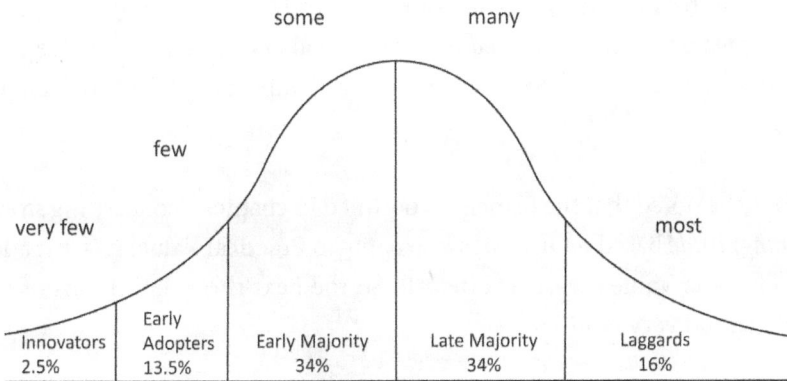

This is one generic template for easily reporting Acceptance Value and Practical Value: "According to the subjective data, this service (or product) is accepted by _____ and/but used by _____." The Acceptance Value result goes in the first blank, and the Practical Value result goes in the second blank.

In our example of valet parking revisited:

$1,600/2,000 \times 100 = 80\%$ (*high* Acceptance Value, $n = 2,000$)
$900/2,000 \times 100 = 45\%$ (*marginal* Practical Value, $n = 2,000$)

The results can now be equally well reported as the following sentence: "The subjective data shows that the service is accepted by *many* and used by *some*." For a professional familiar with value statistics, this sentence should provide just as much information as the following two sentences:

1) "The subjective data shows that the service has *high Acceptance Value* and *marginal Practical Value.*"

2) "The subjective data shows that the service has *Acceptance Value between 50% and 84%* and *Practical Value between 16% and 50%.*"

As increased numbers of questions and groups are analyzed, it helps to use fewer words but consistent language to describe larger amounts of information. The key words are *accepted* for Acceptance Value and *used* for Practical Value. Any reasonable synonyms of these words, such as *adopted/supported* for *accepted* and *utilized/needed* for *used*, are also good choices. Once data is reported regularly in this format, however, it is important to keep the language the same.

It should be noted that the principles outlined in chapter 3 concerning *strength and magnitude* based on n-values also apply to Practical Value. It is just another Consensus Value measure, after all. So the next three definitions of value should sound very familiar.

Definition of Value #8

Total Practical Value = multiple of a subjective Practical Value (in Value Units) and the number of people using (or needing) a product or service

Definition of Value #9

Combined Total Practical Value =
sum of all Total Practical Values
being compared

Definition of Value #10

Collective Practical Value =
Combined Total Practical Value
over maximum Combined Total
Practical Value × 100

The best way to rapidly learn these terms is to work through an example that focuses on the Practical Value component. This example also illustrates why it is considered important to collect subjective data about both Acceptance Value and Practical Value.

As an example, consider an emergency button in the bathroom at the Southern California UFO Club.

The clubhouse bathroom has an emergency button that costs the club $1,000 per month to keep active by paying a monitoring company. State law does not require this service, and the club officers are trying to decide if they should keep it active or not due to financial constraints.

A subjective survey shows these results:
The Star Wars committee has 500 members, 400 of whom support the emergency button. When asked who needs or uses the button, the result was 10 members.

The Star Trek committee has 100 members, 90 of whom support the emergency button. When asked who needs or uses the button, the result was 2 members. The Quantum Leap committee has 100 members, 100 of whom support the emergency button. When asked who needs or uses the button, the result was 60.

Without generating all the formal numbers, it is clear to see that all groups consider this service to have *very high* Acceptance Value. The Practical Value also shows a clear trend, but the higher need or utilization number in the Quantum Leap committee warrants a formal evaluation of the situation.

First, determine the subjective Practical Value (and corresponding percentages) for each subgroup and display the n-value:
The Star Trek committee has *very low* Practical Value for this service (2%, $n = 100$).
The Star Wars committee has *very low* Practical Value for this service (2%, $n = 500$).
The Quantum Leap committee has *high* Practical Value for this service (60%, $n = 100$).

Next, calculate the Total Practical Value for each group by assigning Value Units for each subjective score category (very high = 5, high = 4, marginal = 3, low = 2, very low = 1) and multiplying by the n-value:
The Star Trek committee: $1 \times 100 = 100$
The Star Wars committee: $1 \times 500 = 500$
The Quantum Leap committee: $4 \times 100 = 400$

Finally, determine the Collective Practical Value by dividing the Combined Total Practical Value by the maximum Combined Total Practical Value:

$100 + 500 + 400 = 1,000$ (Combined Total Practical Value)

$1,000/3,500 = 28.6\%$ (Collective Practical Value)

Referring to the Rogers' curve, this would fall into the subjective Practical Value category of "marginal."

This could be reported to the club as: "The bathroom button service is supported by *most* members and utilized or needed by *some*."

Since the Practical Value for this service did not fall into the "low" or "very low" categories, the club officers may not want to discontinue the service until they finish surveying the rest of the club.

5
SENTIMENTAL-MYTHOLOGICAL VALUE

"Public sentiment is everything. With public sentiment
nothing can fail."—Abraham Lincoln

A retired professional football player was interviewed by a sports reporter. He
was asked, *"So, what in your living room is valuable to you?"* The football player
answered, *"That jersey over there in the frame is worth $10,000. That old foot-
ball over there in the case is from when I was in high school. It's not worth much,
but it has a lot of **sentimental value** to me."*

Is the football valuable? Of course the answer is yes, but in what way? How much
value does it have? As we continue our discussion of subjective value, the concept of sentimental or mythological value enters the picture. Taking a peek at the
Merriam-Webster dictionary helps frame what kind of value we are looking for:

Sentimental = *b: resulting from feeling rather than reason or thought*
Mythological = *lacking factual basis or historical validity*

These definitions help us further define the type of value we are talking about. The value the player sees in his old high school football is a result of feeling (not reason) and is likely "lacking factual basis." What this really means is that this is the **most subjective** of all Consensus Value measures. An appraiser could say *objectively* that the football is old, broken, and *worthless*. The player will say that it is *priceless* because it reminds him of a time when he was on top of the world. The player's wife may say that it is *worth a little* because it reminds her of some good times in high school.

What is quite interesting about Sentimental-Mythological Value is that while it is "more tainted" (i.e., more subjective), it is also arguably more powerful than either Acceptance Value or Practical Value. This is because Sentimental-Mythological Value involves an imaginary component that by definition does not follow reason or factual basis. This somewhat "magical" value, when measured, does provide some critically important information. It predicts how much a product or service will *enhance the reputation* of a group, company, or organization.

If a service or product carries high Sentimental-Mythological Value in a group, then those people are likely to think of the organization that provides the service or product as being "somehow, unexplainably, deep-down" better than others.

Definition of Value #11

Sentimental-Mythological Value = the number of people who believe a product or service is special or unexplainably valuable, enhancing the reputation of those who provide the service or product (scored as a percentage and reported as a subjective term)

When querying for Sentimental-Mythological Value, the questions should be simple and straightforward. Example questions would include these:

1) Do you think this service makes the organization special in some way compared to similar organizations?
2) Do you think this service makes the organization unique in a good way compared to similar organizations?
3) Do you this service separates this organization in a good way from other similar organizations?

A key similarity with the other Consensus Value measures is that the *strength and magnitude* calculations based on *n*-values presented in chapter 3 also apply to Sentimental-Mythological Value analyses. Therefore, the next three definitions of value are predictable:

Definition of Value #12

Total Sentimental-Mythological Value = multiple of a subjective Sentimental-Mythological Value (in Value Units) and the number of people who feel a product or service is special

Definition of Value #13

Combined Total Sentimental-Mythological Value = sum of all Total Sentimental-Mythological Values being compared

Definition of Value #14

Collective Sentimental-Mythological
Value = Combined Total Sentimental-
Mythological Value over maximum
Combined Total Sentimental-
Mythological Value × 100

As alluded to earlier, a key difference in working with this particular type of subjective data, however, is that the question being asked is, "How does this product or service affect the reputation of the organization?" Acceptance Value and Practical Value analysis is focused on determining how many members of a group value and need/use a particular service or product, not how the value held by members for a service/product reflects on the organization as a whole (i.e., the focus of Sentimental-Mythological Value). This influences how standardized language needs to be presented for Sentimental-Mythological Value reporting.

Using standard language in place of value-statistics language when reporting Sentimental-Mythological Value results continues a familiar, consistent pattern with only slight modification:

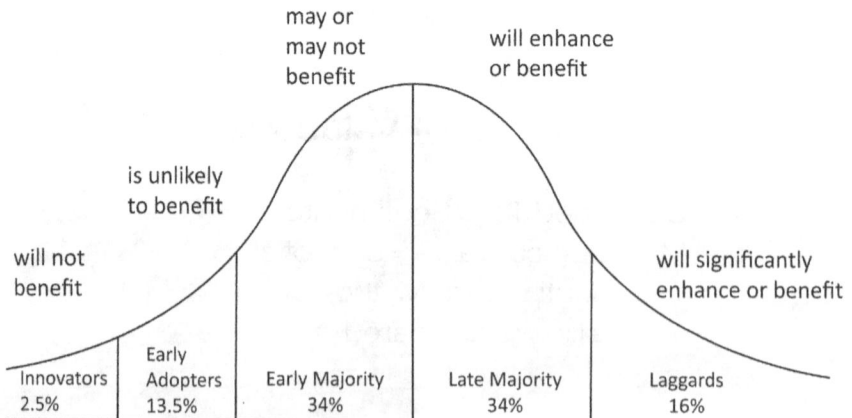

may or
may not
benefit

will enhance
or benefit

is unlikely
to benefit

will not
benefit

will significantly
enhance or benefit

Innovators	Early Adopters	Early Majority	Late Majority	Laggards
2.5%	13.5%	34%	34%	16%

A standard template for reporting Sentimental-Mythological Value would read: "According to the subjective data, this service (or product) _____ the reputation of the organization." The standard Sentimental-Mythological language is inserted in the blank.

Adding more information to the initial Southern California UFO Club example:

When the 2,000 members of the group were surveyed, the final question asked was, "Does the NASA Curiosity Mars Rover live-stream service make the SC UFO Club *special in some way* compared to similar clubs?" On the survey, 1,700 members replied yes to this question.

Performing a simple calculation shows $1,700/2,000 \times 100 = 85\%$
As 85% is above the threshold for "very high" subjective score, the club officers can consider the live-stream service having *very high* Sentimental-Mythological Value. If the Acceptance Value and Practical Value are also high, this means the service is not just accepted and utilized/needed, but the service is also actively enhancing or increasing the reputation of the club. With all this subjective information, it would seem foolish to stop the service unless the club officers are prepared to face some disappointed members and possibly negative word-of-mouth criticism. If all three Consensus Value components were *very high*, the official report could read: "The subjective data shows that the service is accepted by *most* members, utilized or needed by *most* members, and *will significantly enhance or benefit* the reputation of the club."

6

STRATEGIC CONSENSUS VALUE

"Consensus isn't just about agreement."—David Graeber

If the goal is to keep a subjective analysis simple, the questions should still include Acceptance Value and Practical Value queries as a minimum. After performing these calculations a few times, however, many value-statistics professionals would probably not feel burdened by adding the Sentimental-Mythological Value component. When subjective value calculations contain Acceptance Value, Practical Value, and Sentimental-Mythological Value queries together, some strategic decision making can occur.

After collecting subjective data for all three Consensus Value components, it is sometimes useful to take a step back and look at the whole picture. Usually the purpose of this type of "satellite view" is to decide whether a product or service has enough value within a group to keep it. Rather than a detailed debate about Acceptance Value versus Practical Value, sometimes organizations just want to decide *yes* or *no* on specific products or services. Since key "yes or no decisions" are also frequently referred to as "strategic decisions," the term Strategic Consensus Value can be applied to this subjective data analysis methodology.

Definition of Value #15

Strategic Consensus Value =
subjective measures that contain
Acceptance Value, Practical Value,
and Sentimental-Mythological Value
components (commonly reported as
combined Value Units over maximum
possible combined Value Units x 100)

While the subjective scores for Acceptance Value, Practical Value, and Sentimental-Mythological Value showed a high level of detail (very low, low, marginal, high, very high) based on corresponding percentage scores, the Strategic Consensus Value actually strives for a lower level of detail.

When deciding strategically whether to keep a product or service, the Rogers' curve can be viewed more simply by drawing a dividing line at the 50% mark. This curve helps to answer the question: "Should the product or service be continued?"

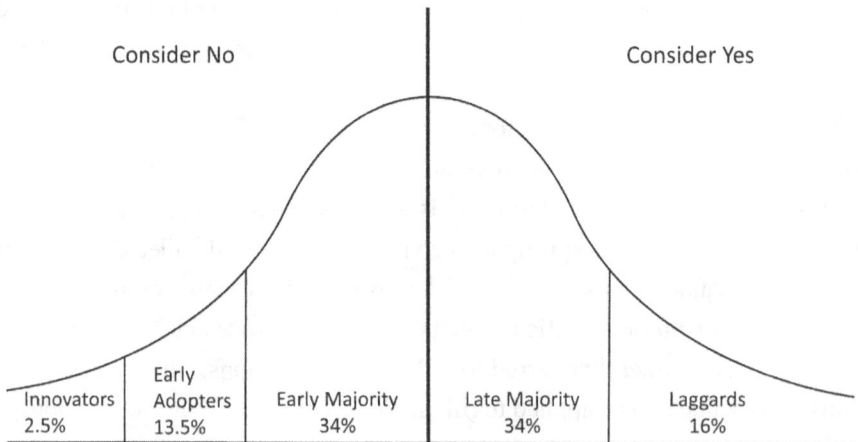

| | Consider No | | | Consider Yes |

| Innovators 2.5% | Early Adopters 13.5% | Early Majority 34% | Late Majority 34% | Laggards 16% |

This also helps simplify analyzing all components of subjective value. A useful template involves assigning Value Units to each subjective value measure. Imagine a grid that shows all three Consensus Value elements. This is called a Strategic Consensus Value Chart:

Acceptance Value	1	2	3	4	5
Practical Value	1	2	3	4	5
Sentimental Value	1	2	3	4	5

Using all the techniques described in previous chapters, subjective data can be converted to Value Units in order to describe how much value a group holds for a product/service and in what way this value may affect the organization's reputation. Since all the value measures are in Value Units, additional calculations can be performed.

For the sake of simplicity, it is better to start by looking at a single group, that way strength and magnitude calculations do not need to be shown.

Remember, in our example from chapter 1, the Southern California UFO Club has 2,000 members. When surveyed, 1,800 members noted that they supported the club's provided live data stream of NASA's Curiosity Mars Rover project.

When asked if they used or needed the service, 300 replied yes.
When the 2,000 members of the group were surveyed, the final question asked was, "Does the NASA Curiosity Mars Rover live-stream service make the SC

SFO Club *special in some way* compared to similar clubs?" On the survey, 1,700 members replied yes to this question.

The club officers are wondering whether or not to keep this service going since there does not seem to be that many members who use the service.

Performing a few simple calculations shows the following:
1,800/2,000 × 100 = 90% *very high* Acceptance Value
300/2,000 × 100 = 15% *low* Practical Value
1,700/2,000 × 100 = 85% *very high* Sentimental-Mythological Value

This can be described in Value Units as follows:
5 Value Units of Acceptance Value
2 Value Unit of Practical Value
5 Value Units of Sentimental-Mythological Value

The Strategic Value Chart easily shows this service's strengths and weaknesses:

Acceptance Value	1	2	3	4	5
Practical Value	1	2	3	4	5
Sentimental Value	1	2	3	4	5

Since the decision to keep the live data stream of NASA's Curiosity Mars Rover project is ultimately a yes or no question, a Strategic Consensus Value needs to be calculated.

The total number of Value Units for all three Consensus Value elements is
5 (Acceptance Value) + 2 (Practical Value) + 5 (Sentimental-Mythological
Value) = 12 Value Units

Dividing this by the maximum possible Value Units gives us a Strategic
Consensus Value, displayed here as a percentage:

$12/15 \times 100 = 80\%$

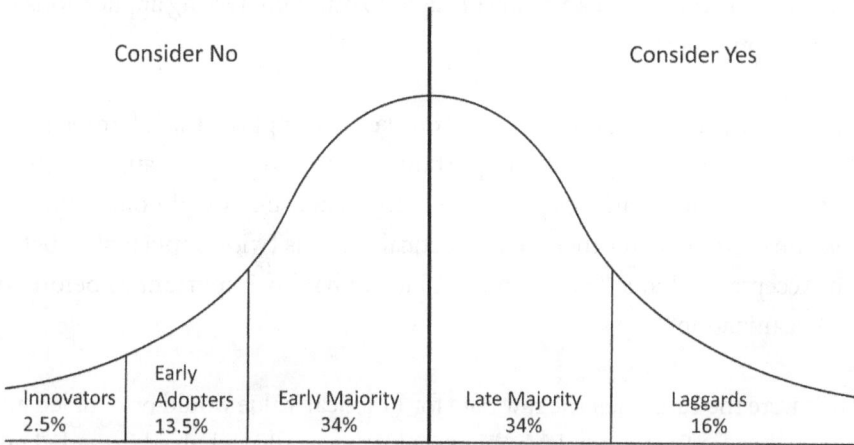

| Innovators 2.5% | Early Adopters 13.5% | Early Majority 34% | Late Majority 34% | Laggards 16% |

Consider No   Consider Yes

Referring to the Rogers' curve shows us that this service is clearly on the "consider yes" side of the curve. In a simplified world, a decision could simply be
made based on this analysis. Individual organizations may choose to set a
threshold where the answer is always "yes, continue the service" or "no, discontinue the service." This would be at the discretion of the organization's
leadership (hence this is strategic decision making).

One possible way to use this analysis is as follows:

1) If the total Value Units are 7 or fewer, discontinue the service.
2) If the total Value Units are 8 or more, continue the service.

A more prudent way to use this analysis is the following:

1) If the total Value Units are 10 or greater, continue the service.

2) If the total Value Units are 6 or fewer, discontinue the service.
3) If the total Value Units are 7, 8, or 9, a vote is needed.

There are many possibilities for how to use this data. Ultimately, this type of subjective analysis is merely trying to get a sense for how the group feels about a specific service or product. Listing all the possible strategic uses for Consensus Value measures is beyond the scope of this text, but hopefully introducing the concept has already brought to mind interesting applications for subjective analyses.

All these calculations, however, make one key assumption: that all three forms of subjective value are equally important. Without trying to cause too much confusion, a value-statistics professional may choose to weight one subjective measure more than another (i.e., "Practical Value is twice important as before and Acceptance Value/Sentimental Value are half as important as before for this organization").

If this were the case, then the raw data for Practical Value would be doubled and the raw data for Sentimental-Mythological Value would be halved (rounded up). The previous example's Strategic Data Chart would therefore look like this:

Acceptance Value	1	2	3	4	5
Practical Value	1	2	3	4	5
Sentimental Value	1	2	3	4	5

The total Value Unit count is now 3 + 4 + 3 = 10

This may or may not influence decision making for this specific organization. The score is still on the "consider yes" side of the curve but much closer to the middle. The strategic rules made by the organization now come into play. The effects of assigning Value Units to a range of percentages are now more noticeable. A product or service that has marginal scores in all three Consensus Value categories, for example, would still achieve 9 Value Units. As such, value-statistics professionals should look at the individual measures as well to get a better overall sense for the value held by a group for the product or service. A conservative organization, for example, may choose to round the Value Unit scores down rather than up. If more specific and accurate subjective data is needed, the Value Unit scale can be adjusted (a detailed discussion about this can be found in chapter 9).

Since people in a group may be asked about anything, the number of topics that can be evaluated for Strategic Consensus Value is practically infinite. This explains why these types of value measurements are so useful, even if they are affected by the limitations of subjective data. Fascinating insights can be gained by adding these types of value assessments to objective value measures. Both simple and complex topics can be evaluated. In order to wrap up our primary discussion of Consensus Value-based subjective data analysis, let us walk through a Strategic Consensus Value evaluation for two everyday topics.

Let us approach a new example—paper money.
In California, 10,000 people were asked three basic questions about a $10 bill (paper money):

1) Do you think this $10 bill is valuable?
2) Would you use this $10 bill?
3) Do you think there is anything special about this $10 bill when compared to other bills?

Results of the survey:
9,000/10,000 people felt the $10 bill was valuable.
9,900/10,000 people felt they would use the $10 bill.
100/10,000 people felt that the $10 bill was special compared to other bills.

Now let us add one objective data element: the rectangular piece of cloth with ink on it that is the $10 bill itself costs about $0.05 to make. The $10 bill has little physical value. This just gives a basic example of how subjective data can be used next to objective value to gain insight about a product or service.

The following is a basic subjective value report for the $10 bill:

The $10 bill has very high Acceptance Value (90%, $n = 10,000$).

The $10 bill has very high Practical Value (99%, $n = 10,000$).

The $10 bill has very low Sentimental-Mythological Value (1%, $n = 10,000$).

Acceptance Value	1	2	3	4	5
Practical Value	1	2	3	4	5
Sentimental Value	1	2	3	4	5

"The $10 bill is accepted as valuable by *most* people, is used by *most* people, and *will not benefit* the reputation of the government."

This already gives some useful information about the $10 bill. First, most people in this group think it is valuable and useful (even though the objective data shows that the physical value is very little). That is good for the government. If the Acceptance Value or Practical Value were low, that could signify a big problem. Second, the Sentimental-Mythological Value is very low. This means people do not think it particularly special in any way. Since money does not need to generate sentimental value per se, this is not a big problem. Having an "overall" subjective value measure would still be useful.

Therefore, what is the Strategic Consensus Value of the $10 bill within this group?

As there is only one group of people being queried, each subjective value score (very high, very high, and very low) can be assigned a Value Unit as introduced in chapter 3.

Strategic Consensus Value = 11/15 × 100 = 73%

Based on this basic analysis, there would be no reason to change the $10 bill unless the government wanted to increase its Sentimental-Mythological Value. Increasing the Sentimental-Mythological Value would mean making the $10 bill special in some way. This might be accomplished by changing the design, color, or even scent of the bill.

For another example, let us consider nuclear weapons.
10,000 people in California were asked three basic questions about nuclear weapons in the United States:
1) Do you think nuclear weapons are a good thing?
2) Do you feel that we will need or use nuclear weapons?
3) Do you think there is anything special about nuclear weapons that makes the Unite States better than other countries?

Results of the survey are as follows:
6,000/10,000 people felt that nuclear weapons were a good thing.
1,000/10,000 people felt that nuclear weapons were needed or would be used.
9,000/10,000 people felt that nuclear weapons made the United States special in some way.

Now let us add one objective data element: the physical value of an average nuclear weapon is about $100,000,000. A nuclear weapon has extremely high physical value.

A basic subjective value report for nuclear weapons would be as follows:
Nuclear weapons have high Acceptance Value (60%, $n = 10,000$).
Nuclear weapons have low Practical Value (10%, $n = 10,000$).

Nuclear weapons have very high Sentimental-Mythological Value (90%, $n = 10{,}000$).

Acceptance Value	1	2	3	4	5
Practical Value	1	2	3	4	5
Sentimental Value	1	2	3	4	5

"Nuclear weapons are accepted as valuable by *many* people, are felt to be needed by *a few* people, and *will significantly benefit* the reputation of the government."

This provides some useful information about nuclear weapons. First, many people in this group think nuclear weapons are valuable, but the tally is much more mixed than with the $10 bill. That is good for the government since they are spending $100,000,000 on each of these weapons. Few people actually think the weapons are needed or will be used, however. This means that if something were to reduce the Acceptance Value for nuclear weapons (e.g., if the price increased to $1,000,000,000 per unit), the government would need to be prepared to justify the expenditure. Fortunately for the government, the Sentimental-Mythological Value is extremely high for nuclear weapons, which means that this group thinks there is something special or magical about them. This may explain why the Acceptance Value is so high for a product/service that has low Practical Value.

Therefore, what is the Strategic Consensus Value within this group for nuclear weapons?

As there is only one group of people being queried, each subjective value score (high, low, very high) can be assigned a Value Unit as introduced in chapter 3.

Strategic Consensus Value = $11/15 \times 100 = 73\%$

Based on the basic analysis, the government would not need to significantly consider discontinuing this product/service. The government may want to continue to monitor the subjective value of the product/service, however, as any major decrease in Acceptance Value or Sentimental-Mythological Value may result in this product/service being challenged.

7
THE VALUE EQUATION

"There is no value in life except what you choose
to place upon it..."—Henry David Thoreau

This chapter is dedicated to explaining *the* Value Equation. The emphasis is on the "*the*." There is only one central Value Equation. There can be many variants of this equation that can be called Value Formulas (discussed in the next chapter). **The most important concept to understand is that the Value Equation is not primarily used for doing mathematics** (that is the purpose of Value Formulas). *The* Value Equation defines how objective value and some subjective value is created. **The Value Equation is a *vetting* equation used to *predict* if a product or service will create value.**

Definition of Value #16

The Value Equation

$$V = \frac{Q}{\text{Cost}}$$

Value equals "big Q" Quality over Cost. Big Q Quality can have many elements ("little q" elements). It is often necessary to look at what kind of "little q" elements are being analyzed as the units may not match. Cost is the literal monetary cost for that product or service. Although Cost has a universal unit (money, currency), it can still be broken down into "little c" cost components if desired.

The importance of *the* Value Equation as a vetting equation is that it plays a part in showing why all forms of increased quality, together or combined, and all forms of decreased cost, individually or combined, can equal increased value.

The key concept can be broken down as such:
If:

1) Increased q1 ("little q" quality) = increased value
2) Increased q2 = increased value
3) Increased q3 = increased value
4) Decreased c1 ("little c" cost) = increased value
5) Decreased c2 = increased value
6) Decreased c3 = increased value

$$\uparrow V = \uparrow Q$$
$$\uparrow V = \downarrow C$$

Then:

By Euclid's Axiom of Transitive Property of Equality:

q1, q2, q3, c1, c2, and c3 can all = value (together or individually)

$$\uparrow V = \uparrow Q + \downarrow C$$

Conclusion:

Both Quality and Cost can be measured to determine value, but both components are not necessarily needed together to create value (if a counter variable is constant). Measuring Quality alone can be used to demonstrate value creation. Measuring Cost alone can be used to demonstrate value creation. Measuring Quality and Cost together can be used to demonstrate value creation.

$$\Delta V = \Delta Q + \Delta C$$

A value-statistics professional must be able to measure value creation from a Quality-only perspective, a Cost-only perspective, and a Quality-Cost perspective. In addition, Euclid's Axiom tells us that there must be a value where some little q's and little c's are equal. Moreover, all little q's and little c's must be describable in some form of Value Unit that can be combined in a logical way. See the end of the following "Quality" section for an example of a *direct conversion from an increased quality measure to a cost savings measure.* A very basic introduction to using Value Units for non-Consensus Value subjective analysis is also presented later in this chapter.

Quality

The "big Q" Quality contains *anything* an organization considers to increase quality. Therefore *every* "little q" quality component of Quality has already been *vetted* by the organization. In addition, each "little q" quality component can by itself or in any combination create value by increasing Quality.

In health care a common list of Quality components ("little q" components) would be as follows:
  1) Outcomes (objective)
  2) Outcomes (subjective—patient/family reported)
  3) Access to care (objective)
  4) Appropriateness (objective)
  5) Medical record quality (objective)
  6) Patient satisfaction (subjective)

As each of these subcategories can be quite involving when it comes to value-statistics analysis, most organizations must initially focus on a few select "little q" components. If more than one is being measured simultaneously, then the value potential can simply be vetted as if the "little q" elements were summed together following the model of *the* Value Equation. This is the most basic variant of *the* Value Equation but still just represents a vetting equation.

$$V = \frac{q1 + q2 + q3}{c1 + c2 + c3}$$

When just looking at a quality component alone, Euclid's Axiom shows us that value can be created of its own accord. This does not, however, guarantee that quality initiatives will not affect cost as they are bound by the logic of *the*

Value Equation. As such, organizations need to make a local decision as to whether or not a "cost balance measure" is needed. As alluded to earlier, the main difficulty arises if **there are different units for each "little q" component.** This is one reason mastering the creation of Value Unit scales is important for a value-statistics professional (see chapter 9). Even more challenging is the fact that quality data may be *objective or subjective*. Working with objective measures is easier, but as Euclid's Axiom shows us, the subjective measures cannot be ignored if it fits a quality component of *the* Value Equation. More on this later.

This example relates to quality increases:
A health care organization wants to improve the quality of patient charts by placing an obesity code on the problem list of all patients with BMI (body mass index) greater than 30. As the organization has an electronic medical record, this can be done automatically and help get patients to classes or services more efficiently if desired. As there is no predictable cost associated with this action, value can be measured directly by analyzing the quality improvement of patient charts (with cost held constant by assumption).

This example *assumes that no cost was incurred* by the project/action. It shows how value can be created purely by measuring quality. It does not, however, show how quality improvement may be equivalent to some amount of cost reduction. This is yet another principle of value creation shown to be theoretically possible by Euclid's Axiom.

Quality improvement must be able to equal some amount of cost reduction. Thus, here is how this works out in our example:
If the obesity code project instantly added 10,000 obesity codes to appropriate charts, hence identifying 10,000 more obese patients, the quality of the medical record has been improved as measured by "updated charts." Conversion to a direct cost measure may be quite difficult but has already been shown to be possible via Euclid's Axiom.

Conversion factors can be made using some publically available sources.

Centers for Disease Control and Prevention, FastStats, Obesity and Overweight
Centers for Disease Control and Prevention, maps of diabetes and obesity 1994, 2000, 2010
US Census, population data 1994
"The economic impact of obesity in the United States", Ross A Hammond, Ruth Levine, Washington, DC, Economic Studies Program, Brookings Institute 3 (August 2010): 285-295

In this example, 1994 data from the Centers for Disease Control, the US Census, and the Brookings Institute can be used to create a conversion factor. At that time the population of the United States was about 265,000,000. Around 18% of this population was obese, or 47,700,000 people. The economic impact to health insurance for obesity was 7.7 billion dollars, or $161/patient/year.

Now some local data from the medical group can be introduced. It is known that about 5% of all obese patients are referred to weight loss programs in the group and that 75% of those patients lose significant weight (enough to drop from obesity to low overweight or normal weight).

Now there is enough information to convert the pure quality unit of "updated charts" to a cost reduction amount. Of the 10,000 newly identified patients, it is predicted that 5%—or 500 patients—will be referred to weight loss programs. Of those 500 patients, 75%—or 375 patients—will lose significant weight. These patients (using a 1994 data conversion value) would represent (375 × $161/patient/year), a total cost of care reduction of $60,375 for the year.

Euclid's Axiom therefore shows us that a quality improvement of 10,000 obesity codes added to a chart (q1) can equal a cost reduction of $60,375 (c1) for the year in this particular example.

This is admittedly quite complicated and tedious with multiple levels of assumptions. A simpler way to look at quality and cost clearly is needed. As will be seen later, Value Units provide a critical simplification option for the value calculation process. The key point here is that cost calculations can be held to the logic of the Value Equation and Euclid's Axiom of Transitive Property of Equality.

Cost

When it comes to *the* Value Equation, the Cost component is the easiest to work with. Cost data is practically always objective (facts rather than opinions). Whether it is the same project or multiple projects, measuring a reduction in cost to increase value will always involve monetary units. Even if you are using different currencies per project, they can easily be converted to the same unit. Early value creation projects may want to start by measuring monetary savings as this is often the easiest data to obtain, manipulate, and report. As will be presented later, conversion of cost measures to Value Units is also more straightforward. The same counter-assumption is made when working with the cost component alone: value can be created, but this does not guarantee that quality will not be affected. As such, organizations need to make a local decision as to whether or not a "quality balance measure" is needed. The purpose and logic behind balance measures is explained thoroughly in the next chapter.

Now let us turn to a cost reduction example:
A health care organization is going to make prephysical examination forms available to patients on the Internet. Since the organization already has server space for it, a full IT team, and the form design, the cost of implementing the program is negligible. As many patients use the online portal, it is expected to attract a fair amount of interest. This will significantly reduce costs by

eliminating the need for paper forms. As the paper forms are available anyway if the patients want them, there is no predicted negative effect against quality. As such, value will be measured directly by cost reduction (*with quality held constant by assumption*).

Introduction to Advanced Concepts (Subjective Data and *the* Value Equation)

Recall that *the* Value Equation is primarily used to measure objective data. Some subjective elements, however, can increase value via *the* Value Equation. As all of the previous chapters discussed subjective data, we will begin with a subjective data introductory example. This subjective data is quite different, however, than the subjective data discussed earlier in the book. The simplest way to measure value for a product or service using subjective data is to set a Value Unit scale based on the Rogers's curve and utilize basic questions as outlined in chapters 2–5. When this "direct" form of value measurement is not used, value from subjective data can still be measured via the Value Equation.

Subjective data in a format that cannot be used to determine Consensus Value falls into the Quality component of *the* Value Equation. There are many important forms of subjective data within health care, for example, that would need to be measured via *the* Value Equation. These would include the following:

1) Patient reported outcomes (PROs)
2) Family/third party reported outcomes (F3Os)
3) Patient satisfaction

This type of subjective data perfectly illustrates the importance of *the* Value Equation as a vetting equation. In the upcoming example *the* Value Equation does not need to be used for mathematical calculations.

Here is a patient reported outcome example for creating a simple Value Unit scale and performing basic data interpretation:

A patient reported outcome might include the amount of days a patient had moderate-severe pain after a surgery (as measured by a survey). Having fewer days of pain after a surgery clearly increases the quality of the service when vetted by *the*

Value Equation. In this case the data will be subjective (a survey completed by the patient and measuring opinion). The questions will not be about Consensus Value, so a basic analysis using a Rogers' curve Value Units scale cannot be considered. So a new Value Unit scale needs to be created to convert the subjective data to Value Units (feel free to read ahead in chapter 9 if you desire a deeper understanding of Value Units at this time). Recognize that creating a Value Formula to perform mathematical calculations is not always needed even though *the* Value Equation is needed to determine if this measure would increase value or not.

In this example we will use the following raw data (assuming three different surgeons):
Following hip replacement surgery, the number of postoperative days in moderate-severe pain (pain scale 7–10/10):

4 days in moderate to severe pain: 10 patients
5 days in moderate to severe pain: 5 patients
6 days in moderate to severe pain: 10 patients
7 days in moderate to severe pain: 20 patients
8 days in moderate to severe pain: 10 patients
9 days in moderate to severe pain: 5 patients
10 days in moderate to severe pain: 5 patients

As the number of days in moderate to severe pain ranges from 4 days to 10 days, a reasonable Value Unit scale might be as follows:

Number of Days in Moderate to Severe Pain

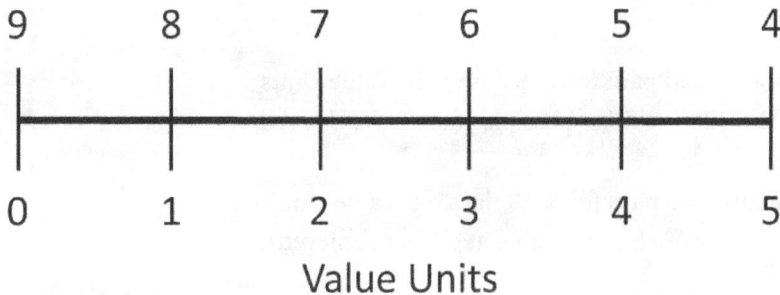

9	8	7	6	5	4

0	1	2	3	4	5

Value Units

This scale can be used much like the Rogers' curve scale. With this scale, some basic value calculations can be performed on the subjective data. If we look at this data as one group of "hospital patients," then the total number of patients is 65. Two simple questions about value might be "How much value was generated within this group of patients in regards to postoperative pain control?" and "Is there room for improvement?" Since these questions are asking not only for measurement of value but possibly some interpretation as well, logic or research must also be attached to the scale. (Recall that the Rogers' curve already has an inherent logic built into it.) **It is at this point where some additional clinical information is needed if any interpretation is to be done.** If the hip-replacement team (which may include surgeons, staff, and patients) determined that having a patient out of moderate-severe pain within 4–5 days is excellent, 5–8 days is average, and in pain equal to or longer than 9 days is unacceptable, the problem can be solved to a higher level of detail (note this would constitute *a local clinical standard*).

With these statistics, we can calculate a simple answer to the question: "How much value was generated?"

Summation of all Value Units:
70 Value Units + 80 Value Units + 0 Value Units = 150 Value Units

Understanding what this means requires a more detailed answer:

15 patients had pain for 4–5 days = 70 Value Units
70/75 (maximum value possible for 15 patients) × 100 = 93.3% of possible value was achieved

40 patients had pain for 6–8 days = 80 Value Units
80/200 × 100 = 40% of possible value was achieved

10 patients had pain for 9–10 days = 0 Value Units
0/50 × 100 = 0% (i.e., no value at all was achieved)

Total possible Value Units for post-op pain control = 65 × 5 Value Units = 325

Of all the value that could have been generated:
150 Value Units / 325 Value Units = 46%
Only 150 Value Units, or 46% of the possible value, were created.
This could be interpreted as "plenty of room for improvement."

We can also calculate the following based on the local clinical standard:
15/65 × 100 = 23% of patients had excellent care (corresponding to 93.3% of the maximum possible value in this subgroup).
40/65 × 100 = 62% of patients had average care (corresponding to 40% of maximum possible value in this subgroup).
10/65 × 100 = 15% of patients had poor care (corresponding to no value at all). This could be interpreted by the following statement: "High levels of value are generated by excellent pain control."

If the focus of this investigation is value creation, additional analysis can be done to look at other groups, individual surgeons, hospital wards, and so forth. Our example merely introduces the topic of using value measures as part of non-Consensus Value subjective data analysis.

An important point to carry forward is that while measuring value is a key skill, interpreting value measures requires additional logic or definition. *The* Value Equation told us reduced days in pain created value (a subjective Quality measure). The patient reported outcomes survey measured the data to show if value was created. The Value Unit scale allowed us to convert the subjective measures to Value Units, allowing for better interpretation of the data. We could just stop there and measure value over time to create comparisons. The first question simply asked how much value was created, after all. The simplest of answers would have just summed all the Value Units and answered 65. Similar to the interpretation of Consensus Value, we expanded our investigation with an example of how to demonstrate levels of value. If we wish to assign any "grade" of value (high, low, etc.), then the Value Unit scale must also have logic or research built into it. Clinical variation reduction is an example of a methodology used to assign this logic to Value Unit scales following creation of a clinical standard. While standard variation statistics will be discussed later in this book, the specific philosophy behind clinical variation reduction will not be detailed. (See L. Shapiro, *Quality Care, Affordable Care, 2013*, for more information about clinical variation reduction.)

It should be noted that *the* Value Equation as it applies to health care is quite similar to the "marketing" Value Equation.

Definition of Value #17

The "marketing" Value Equation

$$V = \frac{\text{Benefit}}{\text{Cost}}$$

This is just something to keep in mind as all quality improvement projects should result in a benefit for the patient. It is a useful "double check" to see if the quality being generated really is a benefit to the patient.

8

VALUE FORMULAS AND TIERED VALUE CREATION

"However beautiful the strategy, you should occasionally look at the results."—Winston Churchill

After vetting whether or not a product or service will generate value, some data needs to be collected. While *the* Value Equation **predicts** if value *will be created*, Value Formulas are used to **measure** if value *is being created*. Any formula based on the logic of *the* Value Equation is referred to as a **Value Formula**. As mentioned in the previous chapter, if a formula measures quality in order to study value creation, there may be effects on cost. Conversely, if a formula measures cost, there may be an effect on quality.

Just as Consensus Value calculations can have higher or lower degrees of accuracy depending on the assumptions made and the Value Unit scale settings (see chapter 9 for details), Value Formulas can also be designed to absorb various degrees of assumptions. The simplest Value Formula just measures Quality or Cost. As all components can equal increased value, Euclid's Axiom allows this calculation but also for the largest assumptions and, accordingly, the greatest possible inaccuracies.

Value Formulas produce the *evidence* of value creation. Value Formulas can be used to perform mathematics. They are integrally involved in direct value calculations. Based on *the* Value Equation, these formulas can measure quality, cost, or both. The results or data that come from Value Formulas are called **value measures**. Quality value measures and cost value measures can be converted to Value Units using Value Unit scales. These Value Units can be reported over time to see trends in value creation.

Value creation can be viewed from the perspective of "confidence in measures." In the field of medicine, recommendations follow a standardized scale of "strength." The better the quality of data and analysis, the stronger the recommendation. Value creation follows a similar principal.

Just measuring an increase in quality to increase value, for example, is possible and quite easy. Euclid's Axiom tells us that any increased quality variable can equal value and any decreased cost variable can equal value. As such, just measuring a quality variable or a cost variable can be used to measure value. Take, for example, access to a clinic (an objective quality measure). If patients are getting into a clinic faster, this is improving the quality of the service. This generates positive value. A Value Units scale can be used to convert an access measure, such as third-next-available appointment, into Value Units. This is a direct measure of value.

A single variable measure of value, however, makes the gross assumption that the counter-variable is constant (i.e., cost is the counter-variable of quality). If we are only measuring quality, we are assuming that cost is not changing significantly. In science, assumptions are made all the time. The question that arises is therefore: "What is the strength of the evidence of value creation?" A value measure that only looks at quality would be considered weak, or a "Tier 1," measurement.

Definitions of Value Creation Tiers

Tier 1 value creation (weaker evidence of value creation): Only a quality variable or a cost variable is measured and converted to Value Units. The assumption is made that the counter-variable is constant.

Tier 2 value creation (standard evidence of value creation): One or more quality variables (or one or more cost variables) are measured and converted to Value Units. A single counter-variable is studied as a "balance measure." This provides the most basic evidence that the counter-variable is constant. The "balance measure" may or may not be reported as Value Units but must be shown to be constant.

Tier 3 value creation (strong evidence of value creation): Multiple quality and multiple cost variables are measured, and all components are converted to Value Units.

If a deeper understanding of Value Unit scale creation is desired, please read chapter 9 first. The following examples present some basic information about Value Unit scales in order to show context for the use of Value Formulas and value measures.

Here is an example of Tier 1 value creation:
Local content experts at a medical clinic have created a clinical standard that states urine culture tests are not needed for most uncomplicated urinary tract infection (UTI) patients. This standard will reduce the number of urine cultures ordered and save patients the cost of the test. The data being measured is the cost (charge data) of the urine cultures six months before and after the clinical standard was created.

Value Formula

$$\text{average laboratory cost per patient (objective cost measure)} = \frac{\text{cost of all laboratory tests associated to uncomplicated UTI codes}}{\text{number of patients treated for uncomplicated UTI}}$$

Value Measures

Average laboratory cost of treating uncomplicated UTI per patient six months before and after clinical standard:

Physician	Before Clinical Standard	After Clinical Standard
MD1	$250	$50
MD2	$200	$50
MD3	$250	$100

This data can then be converted to Value Units using a Value Unit scale:

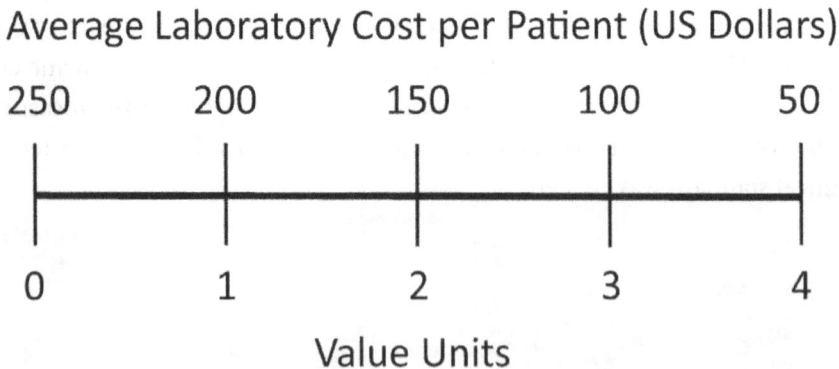

Average Laboratory Cost per Patient (US Dollars)

250	200	150	100	50
0	1	2	3	4

Value Units

Physician	Before Clinical Standard	After Clinical Standard
MD1	0	4
MD2	1	4
MD3	0	3

The data shows that value was created by this clinical standard.

The question that remains unanswered is, "Did this clinical standard negatively affect quality in any way?" As this is a Tier 1 value creation project, the assumption is that the content experts took this into account and that quality is held constant.

Now let us look at an example of Tier 2 value creation:
We will start with the same scenario as example 1 except that this time a "balance measure" was created to look at the number of pyelonephritis (kidney infection) cases six months before and after the clinical standard that followed the initial diagnosis of uncomplicated urinary tract infection. Recall that balance measures may or may not be converted to Value Units (this case just shows a direct data measurement).

Number of pyelonephritis cases following presentation of uncomplicated UTI:

Physician	Before Clinical Standard	After Clinical Standard
MD1	0	0
MD2	0	1
MD3	0	0

The data showed that one case of pyelonephritis occurred after the standard. A chart review of this case showed that the patient actually did not present as an uncomplicated UTI and should have had a urine culture. The reviewers determined this was not the result of the clinical standard but rather clinical decision making. The strong conclusion after review is that the clinical standard did not harm quality based on this measure.

The data now shows value creation by cost reduction and provides stronger evidence that quality is being held constant. As a Tier 2 value creation project, there is now data to support the constancy of the counter-variable (quality).

Now we turn to a Tier 3 example:

The same clinical standard topic will be presented for continuity (uncomplicated UTI treatment). The data being measured this time will include the following:

1) Average cost (charge data) of urine cultures per patient before and after clinical standard
2) Average cost (charge data) of office visit per patient (by level) before and after clinical standard
3) Number of pyelonephritis cases (quality data) before and after clinical standard per 100 cases
4) Number of repeat visits for treatment failure (quality data) before and after clinical standard per 100 cases

Value Formulas

average laboratory cost per patient (objective cost measure) $=$ $\dfrac{\text{cost of all laboratory tests associated to uncomplicated UTI codes}}{\text{number of patients treated for uncomplicated UTI}}$

average cost of office visit for uncomplicated UTI per patient (objective cost measure*) $=$ $\dfrac{\text{cost of all office visits associated to uncomplicated UTI codes}}{\text{number of patients treated for uncomplicated UTI}}$

* Note that in this example, the data will be interpreted as an objective quality measure.

$$\text{number of pyelonephritis cases per 100 uncomplicated UTI cases (objective quality measure)} = \frac{\text{number of clinically verified and charted cases of pyelonephritis within two weeks of uncomplicated UTI code visit and treatment}}{\text{100 patients treated for uncomplicated UTI}}$$

$$\text{number of repeat visits for uncomplicated UTI per 100 cases (objective quality measure)} = \frac{\text{number of clinically verified and charted cases of uncomplicated UTI within two weeks of initial uncomplicated UTI code visit and treatment}}{\text{100 patients treated for uncomplicated UTI}}$$

The clinical standard now includes the additional logic that an uncomplicated UTI should be charged as a level 3 office visit and not higher. The number of pyelonephritis cases and the number of repeat visits will be measured directly as value and not reported as data measures. As such, Value Unit scales will need to be created for these elements:

1) Laboratory cost for treating uncomplicated UTI
2) Office visit cost for treating uncomplicated UTI
3) Number of pyelonephritis cases following uncomplicated UTI diagnosis
4) Number of repeat visits for uncomplicated UTI treatment failure

The first Value Unit scale was seen earlier and shows increasing value as the cost of care goes down. This is a "backward" scale as the smaller cost number corresponds with a higher Value Unit.

Average Laboratory Cost per Patient (US Dollars)

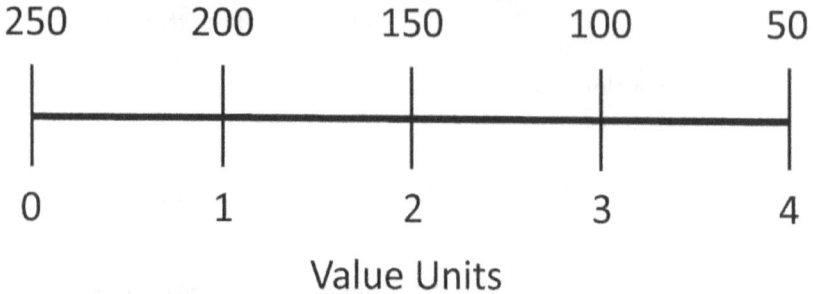

250	200	150	100	50

0	1	2	3	4

Value Units

The second Value Unit scale shows increasing value as cost approaches the correct office visit charge. This is a "crescendo-decrescendo" scale as the Value Units peak at the center of the scale. Note that although cost data is being collected (usually an objective cost measure), this is technically an *objective quality measure* as it is looking for "appropriate office visit billing level."

Average Office Visit Cost per Patient (US Dollars)

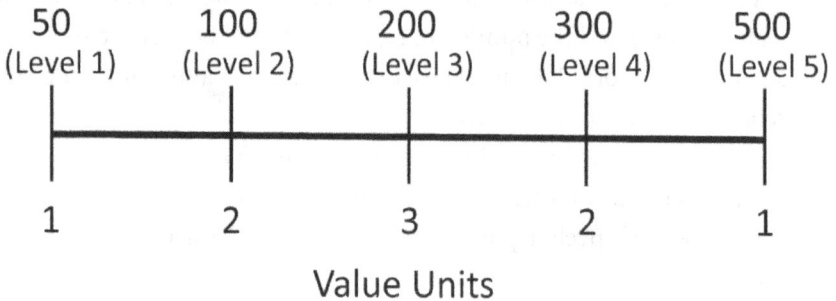

50	100	200	300	500
(Level 1)	(Level 2)	(Level 3)	(Level 4)	(Level 5)

1	2	3	2	1

Value Units

The third Value Unit scale shows increasing value if the number of cases of pyelonephritis per 100 patients is 2 or fewer. The scale shows no value creation if the number of cases of pyelonephritis is greater than 2. This is a "range" scale as the Value Units are assigned to a range of possible numbers.

Number of Pyelonephritis Cases Following Uncomplicated UTI per 100 Cases

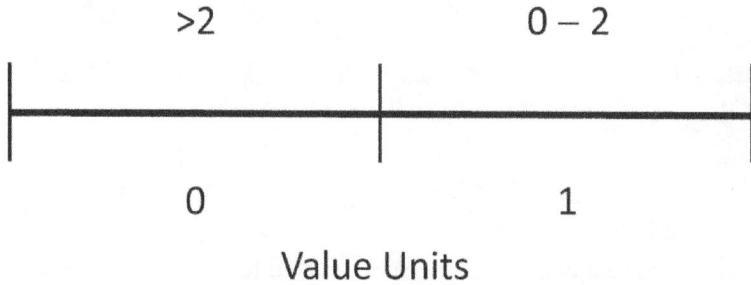

>2   0 – 2

0   1

Value Units

The fourth Value Unit scale shows increasing value if the number of repeat visits to the clinic after treatment for uncomplicated UTI is 0 or 1. The scale shows no value creation if the patient has more than 1 repeat office visit for uncomplicated UTI after treatment. This is also a "range" Value Unit scale.

Number of Repeat Visits Following Uncomplicated UTI per 100 Cases

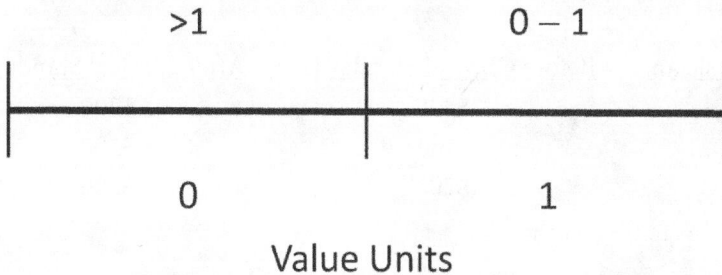

>1   0 – 1

0   1

Value Units

The Value Formulas are now used to generate value measures. The value measures are then converted to Value Units.

Value Formula 1 and Value Unit Scale 1

Raw data for average cost (charge data) of urine cultures per patient before and after clinical standard:

Physician	Before Clinical Standard	After Clinical Standard
MD1	$250	$50
MD2	$200	$50
MD3	$250	$100

The average cost of urine cultures converted to Value Units:

Physician	Before Clinical Standard	After Clinical Standard
MD1	0	4
MD2	1	4
MD3	0	3

Data shows that value was created.

Value Formula 2 and Value Unit Scale 2

Raw data for average cost (charge data by level) of office visit per patient before and after clinical standard:

Physician	Before Clinical Standard	After Clinical Standard
MD1	$300	$200
MD2	$100	$200
MD3	$200	$200

The average cost of office visits converted to Value Units:

Physician	Before Clinical Standard	After Clinical Standard
MD1	2	3
MD2	3	3
MD3	3	3

Data shows that value was created or maintained.

Value Formula 3 and Value Unit Scale 3

Raw data number of pyelonephritis cases (quality data) before and after clinical standard per 100 cases:

Physician	Before Clinical Standard	After Clinical Standard
MD1	0	0
MD2	0	1*(0)
MD3	0	0

* Case review shows that this case was not attributable to the clinical standard and was therefore not counted.

Number of pyelonephritis cases converted to Value Units:

Physician	Before Clinical Standard	After Clinical Standard
MD1	0	1
MD2	0	1
MD3	0	1

Data shows that value was created.

Value Formula 4 and Value Unit Scale 4

Raw data for the number of repeat visits for treatment failure before and after clinical standard per 100 cases:

Physician	Before Clinical Standard	After Clinical Standard
MD1	4	2
MD2	3	1
MD3	3	0

Number of repeat visits converted to Value Units:

Physician	Before Clinical Standard	After Clinical Standard
MD1	0	0
MD2	0	1
MD3	0	1

Data shows that value was created. Note MD1 did not show change.

Clearly Tier 3 value creation requires much more effort. There is more value-statistics work, coordination of data collection, and input of content experts to define Value Unit scales.` There is enough data to report both Tier 2 and Tier 3 value creation. A Tier 2 report would show that value was created by reducing laboratory costs for uncomplicated UTI patients with quality balance measures remaining stable. A Tier 3 report would show that value was created not only by reducing both laboratory costs but also by increasing some quality measures.

A generic "total value" score can also be reported by adding all quality and cost Value Units before and after the clinical standard:

Total Value Units Before Standard	Total Value Units After Standard
8	25

This data can be reported in many formats. Some basic observations would be as such:

1) The Value Units increased from 8 to 25.
2) The Value Units increased threefold.
3) 25 out of a 27 possible Value Units were achieved after starting at a level of 8 Value Units.

Some specific observations:

1) Value measure 1 (cost) increased from 1/12 possible Value Units to 11/12 possible Value Units.
2) Value measure 2 (cost was measured but the results were interpreted as a quality measure) increased from 7/9 possible Value Units to 9/9 possible Value Units.
3) Value measure 3 (quality) increased from 0/3 Value Units to 3/3 possible Value Units.
4) Value measure 4 (quality) increased from 0/3 Value Units to 2/3 possible Value Units.

This simple analysis shows us that the urine culture cost reduction had a dramatic effect on value creation. The quality measures show us that appropriate office visit billing improved, prevention of pyelonephritis was fully achieved and constant, while repeat visits for uncomplicated UTIs still had a little room for improvement.

Some interesting insights are also present in the raw data. Value Formula #2 produced cost data based on office visit charges. Notice that one physician's charges went down, another physician's charges went up, and the third physician's charges stayed the same. Despite these changes in the raw data, value went up or stayed the same for all three physicians. This shows the importance of the Value Unit scale in interpreting the raw data. **Even though one physician's charges increased, his value creation actually went up.** Why is this? This is evident because he was under-coding and not billing accurately for his services. Under-billing can be considered poor-quality documentation or even fraud, so this is an important point. Even though cost data was being measured, *this is technically a quality measure* (selecting the appropriate office visit level). Without the Value Unit scale, this cost data could easily have been misinterpreted.

The key concept to remember is that while Value Formulas are needed to actually measure whether or not value is being created, looking at the raw data itself may not be enough to fully understand if value truly is being created. Value Unit scales are therefore needed to translate the raw value measures into Value Units that can be interpreted easily. The next chapter discusses Value Unit scale creation in more detail.

A final point to be made is that an asterisk (*) should be placed next to a tier level if subjective data is being analyzed alone or with objective data in this manner. *As subjective data is less reliable and prone to unexpected variance, using an asterisk indicator will give a "heads up" to look closer if results appear unusual.* This can simply be written as follows:

"Tier 3* value measures/reports" (includes subjective data) versus "Tier 3 value measures/reports" (only objective data).

9
VALUE UNITS

"Make everything as simple as possible,
but not simpler."—Albert Einstein

As introduced in chapter 3 and demonstrated in chapter 8, Value Units can be thought of as "points" assigned to any value measure that allows mathematics to be performed easier and results to be interpreted more accurately. Sometimes Value Units need to be created in order to have a universal unit, without which any math cannot even be attempted. In reality, Value Units are part of a scale. More specifically, they are the conversion of an objective scale or subjective scale into a Value Unit scale. This allows any objective or subjective measure to be converted to a universal Value Unit so more analysis can be done. It should be noted that this chapter focuses only on the creation of Value Unit scales and not how to perform analyses with Value Units (discussed in chapter 10).

The most basic way of looking at Value Units is as one half of a scale with mirrored units:

Objective Measure

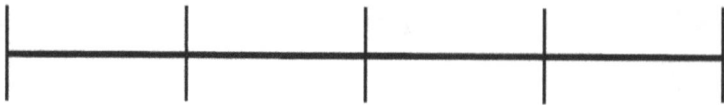

Value Units

OR

Subjective Measure

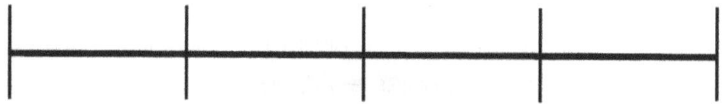

Value Units

If evaluating objective data, the top half of the scale can show any objective measure of Cost or Quality. The lower half of the scale shows the conversion to Value Units. For example, the top half of the scale may show percentage of health care providers compliant to a clinical standard (an objective Quality measure):

Percent Compliance with Clinical Standard

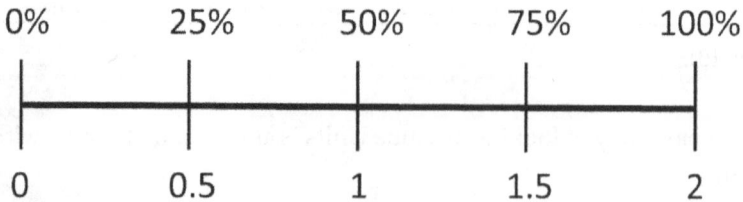

0%	25%	50%	75%	100%
0	0.5	1	1.5	2

Value Units

The bottom half of the scale shows that the assigned Value Units range from 0 to 2. The percentage can now easily be converted to Value Units. **This technique is powerful because both the objective measure scale and the Value Units scale can be changed to fit the requirements of the organization.** In the following example both the objective measure scale and the Value Unit scale have changed:

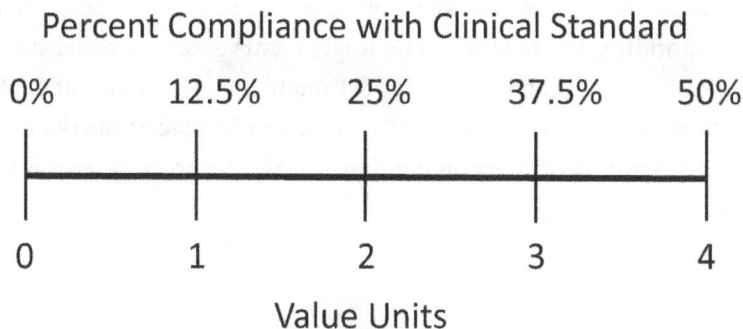

Percent Compliance with Clinical Standard

0%	12.5%	25%	37.5%	50%
0	1	2	3	4

Value Units

The objective scale component can easily be changed to various other measures. The example below shows the number of patients being discharged on time per day from a hospital (an objective Quality measure) being converted to Value Units:

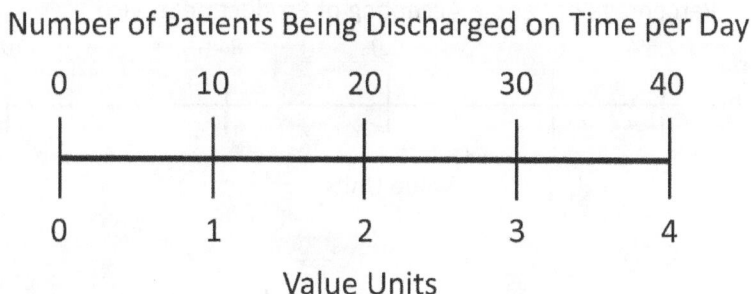

Number of Patients Being Discharged on Time per Day

0	10	20	30	40
0	1	2	3	4

Value Units

The top of the scale can also be a subjective measure as shown earlier in the book with Consensus Value measures. **A second reason Value Unit scales are powerful is that the scale itself (not just the subjective/objective measures and Value Units assigned) can be changed to fit the needs of the organization.** Note that the hypothetical scales shown so far in this chapter have evenly spaced, proportional marks on the scale. There is an equal amount of "space" between percentages (0%, 25%, 50%, etc.) and the corresponding Value Units. The Rogers' curve, on the other hand, has percentage "spaces" that are not proportionate (i.e., first mark at 2.5%, second mark at 16%, third mark at 50%, etc.), so **the placed marks and corresponding Value Units are dependent on the logic or research behind the scale itself.**

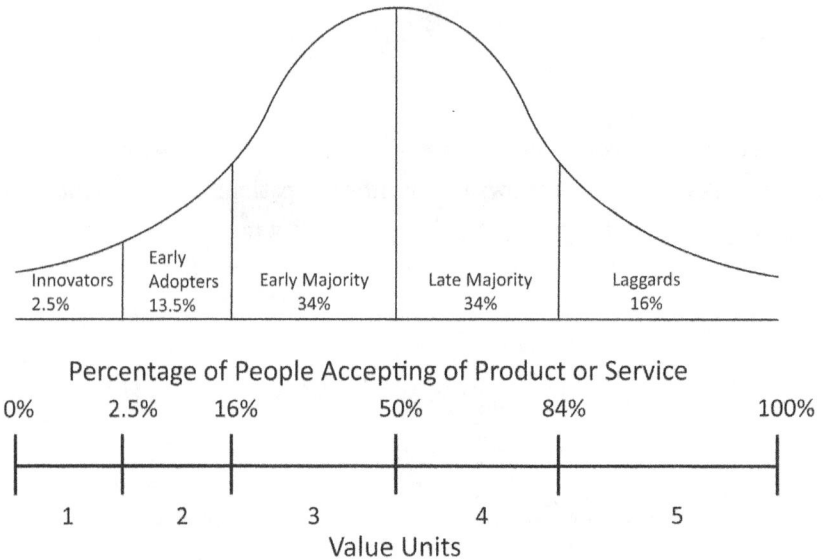

A third reason Value Unit scales are powerful is that the Value Units can be applied to the marks on the scale (threshold limits) or to the spaces between

marks (range limits). Note that on the Rogers' curve–Value Unit scale, the Value Units have been shifted off the marks and into the "range" areas. The Value Units are now not assigned by "threshold" values but rather by any number that falls within the "range." If a value-statistics professional places the Value Unit on a mark, it will create fractional Value Units (i.e., when data passes the threshold, the Value Units will be measured as 1.32 Value Units, for example). If the Value Unit is placed in a range, then the Value Unit is a whole number that corresponds to several possible (fractional) objective/subjective measures. Choosing to assign Value Units to a range makes subsequent value calculations easier (whole numbers) but accepts that there is some variance as to what subjective or objective measure is represented by the Value Unit. Assigning Value Units to a threshold mark increases the accuracy of the reported value score when compared to the subjective/objective measure but makes the resulting value calculations a little more difficult (as the Value Units will now be expressed as fractions or decimals).

As shown in the beginning of the book, Value Units for some subjective analyses (Consensus Values) can be assigned to a *range*. This allows for easier computations to be done. While the Value Units are less accurate than setting them to the *threshold* marks, the resultant information is still useful enough to make informed decisions. As subjective data is less reliable and by definition "tainted," a value-statistics professional may prefer to set the scale in this way to favor ease of calculations. Subjective queries are, after all, trying to gauge the "feel" of a group in regards to a product or service.

Most objective data sets are derived from facts and rely heavily on accuracy to create value via *the* Value Equation logic. Non-Consensus Value subjective data also relies on *the* Value Equation. As such, Value Unit scales set to analyze objective data or non-Consensus Value subjective data should preferentially assign Value Units to the marks as *thresholds*. If simplified reporting is desired, then the results can be set to an "all or nothing" criteria (i.e., a Value Unit is only earned when an objective/subjective measure crosses the *threshold* mark).

When deciding how to "set" the subjective/objective measure and Value Unit scales, a few considerations must be taken into account:
1) Am I analyzing just subjective data?
2) Am I analyzing just objective data?
3) Am I analyzing both subjective and objective data?

Value Unit Scales for Subjective Data Value Calculations

If the value analysis is only looking at subjective data, the simplest approach is to determine Acceptance Value, Practical Value, and Sentimental-Mythological Value. Setting the Value Unit scale depends on a fixed measure scale that can be applied to all three. As the first half of the book demonstrated, an adoption curve, such as the Rogers' curve, nicely fits the requirements of the top of the scale. Since subjective data analysis is trying to determine the value from "feeling" within a group for a product or service, it is acceptable and easier to assign Value Units to a *range* rather than a *threshold*. As there were 5 ranges on the scale Value Units can be assigned to each range in increasing order. Note the logic behind the Value Unit number selection—it is more difficult to obtain a higher percentage of acceptance as defined by the Rogers' curve, and the corresponding ranges should have higher Value Units. Other numbers can be assigned for the Value Units, but again, if the focus is simplicity of calculations, 1–5 works nicely. Once the scale is created, however, it must be held constant for all subjective data calculations. If a higher level of detail and accuracy is demanded for subjective data, then the Value Unit can be set to the marks as *thresholds*. If specific subjective quality data (a.k.a. non-Consensus Value subjective data) needs to be evaluated, then Value Unit scales must be created for each quality measure being evaluated (refer back to chapter 7 for an example details about subjective quality data and *the* Value Equation).

Value Unit Scales for Objective Data Value Calculations

If the value analysis is only looking at objective data, we need to ask these questions:
1) Am I analyzing just cost data?

2) Am I analyzing just quality data (objective data only in this case)?

3) Am I analyzing both cost and quality data?

Value Unit Scales for Objective Cost Value Calculations

When looking at cost data, value is generated via the Value Equation by reducing costs. Since cost has a "natural universal unit" (i.e., money, currency), calculations are fairly straightforward. One rule about Value Unit scales and cost reduction that needs to be taken into account is that the Value Units created by cost reduction have no theoretical maximum (until a product or service is given away for free). As a result, it is quite important to set the Value Unit scale as *user-friendly* as possible. If the goal of an organization is to save $1,000,000 through a project, it would not make much sense to create a scale that makes $1 saved equal to 1 Value Unit. A more reasonable scale might look like the following:

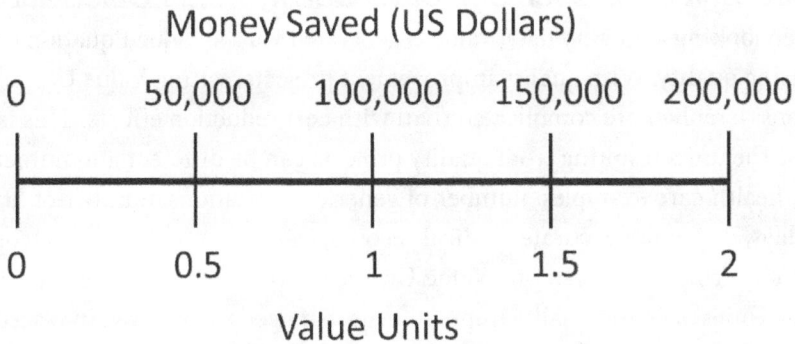

Money Saved (US Dollars)

0	50,000	100,000	150,000	200,000
0	0.5	1	1.5	2

Value Units

A rule of thumb that can be applied to cost reduction value projects is that the Value Unit scale should not set a Value Unit at less than 1% of the total goal. In other words, for the prior example, a Value Unit should be $10,000 saved/reduced or more. If the organization actually thinks the effort will save much more than $1,000,000, a higher Value Unit equivalency needs to be assigned (recall that there is no theoretical maximum for cost savings measures). If the effort saves $5,000,000, for example, and the Value Unit was set to $10,000, the resulting number—500—is quite high. As will be demonstrated later, there is some benefit to trying to set a cost Value Unit scale so that the Value Units that result from predicted measurements end up being at least single digits (See "The Five Golden Steps of Value Unit Scale Creation" in chapter 11). Once a scale is decided upon, however, it needs to be held constant for the entire project. Ideally, if enough information is available to create a reasonable cost Value Scale, then a "universal" scale should be made constant for a project across the entire organization. This scale can be modified to reflect individual subprojects as needed. This methodology is useful in describing value creation for a "snapshot in time"—for example, showing how much cost to the patient was reduced over one year for a specific project. Determining if the value being created by cost savings is sustainable or changing in some important way over time is discussed later.

Value Unit Scales for Objective Quality Value Calculations

When looking at quality data, value is generated via the Value Equation by increasing quality. With quality improvement projects, setting Value Unit scales is considerably more complicated than with cost reduction efforts. This is because the units resulting from quality projects can be different and numerous (i.e., health care examples: number of generic medications, number of hospital days, percent of accurate medical records, interval between colonoscopies, etc.) requiring more than one Value Unit scale to be defined. One rule about Value Unit scales and quality improvement that needs to be taken into account is this: the Value Units created by quality improvement do have a theoretical maximum (when all patients are healthy, when all patients have defect-free care, when all outcomes are favorable, etc.). The first step is to define all "quality categories" accepted or acknowledged within the organization. Recall from chapter 7, for example, a health care organization may define the quality categories as follows:

1) Outcomes (objective)
2) Outcomes (subjective—patient/family reported)

3) Access to care (objective)
4) Appropriateness (objective)
5) Medical record quality (objective)
6) Patient satisfaction (subjective)

Outcomes (Objective)
Outcomes are a popular measure to analyze when it comes to increasing value by increasing quality. The basic principle to keep in mind is that all quality measures, regardless of the unit that comes with the objective data, can be converted to Value Units. As there are many outcome measures that can be studied (see M. E. Porter, *New England Journal of Medicine* 363 [2010]: 2477–2481 for numerous examples) the value-statistics professional must first decide if the analysis will be done on a single outcome data set (single project) or numerous data sets. The true benefit of converting all objective data units to Value Units will be seen in the next chapter. For now, some examples will simply show how Value Unit scales can be created and modified for various data sets.

If the value being measured relates to a single objective outcome measure, the accompanying Value Unit scale is quite easy to define. If the outcomes data, for example, shows that the number of patients being discharged from a hospital ward on time ranges from 10–40, a scale such as this might be generated:

Number of Patients Being Discharged on Time per Day

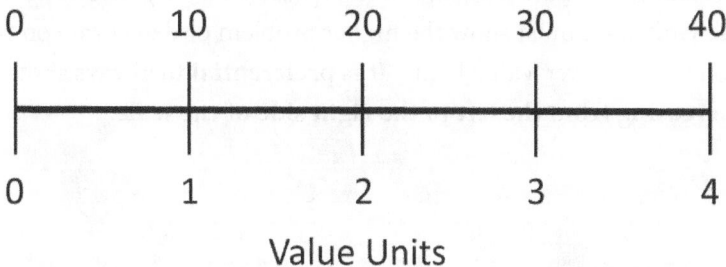

0	10	20	30	40
0	1	2	3	4

Value Units

Note that if the hospital ward only has 40 beds, a result of 40 timely discharges and the corresponding Value Units represents a maximum possible value for this single outcomes measure. If the outcomes measure remains the same (i.e., number of patients being discharged on time per day) but there is a different data source, the Value Unit scale can be changed to accommodate the new data. For example, if there was another hospital ward with 50 beds, and the value-statistics professional wanted to be able to combine or compare Value Units, the previous scale could be extended for the new data set:

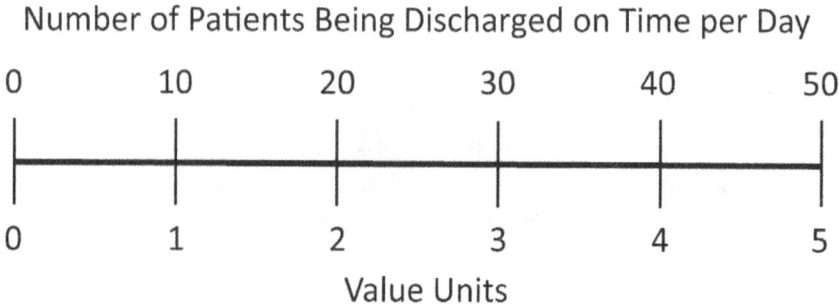

Number of Patients Being Discharged on Time per Day

0	10	20	30	40	50

0	1	2	3	4	5

Value Units

This is the most basic Value Unit scale and is commonly referred to as a "forward" scale. This term is derived from the fact that the numbers on both halves of the scale increase as the scale progresses forward.

If a different outcomes measure is being analyzed, then a new scale needs to be created. If the outcomes measure represents a "negative" effect, then the Value Unit scale must show the higher problem or defect rate on the left corresponding to lower Value Units. **It is preferential to always show Value Units increasing from the left to the right side of the scale**.

Let us look at a new example of another outcomes measure scale showing the number of falls per day on average for Hospital Ward A:

Note that this is a "backward scale" (i.e., the higher objective number is to the left and represents lower Value Units).

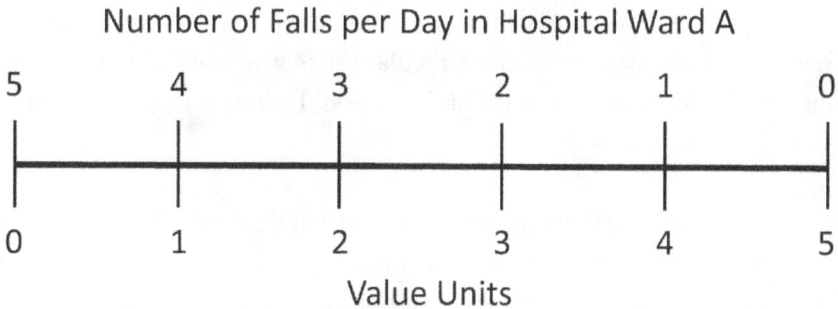

Number of Falls per Day in Hospital Ward A

5	4	3	2	1	0

0	1	2	3	4	5

Value Units

This type of backward scale is needed for "negative" measures that represent harm caused to a patient. A few "positive" measures, however, can use a "backward" Value Unit scale.

Looking at both of the objective outcome measures presented (number of patients discharged on time and number of falls per day), we can do some very basic calculations. Value Units can be added together, compared, and tracked over time; basic variation analysis can be performed; and so forth. This will be shown in detail later. **The basic concept illustrated here is that regardless of whether the data measures a "positive" objective outcome measure (i.e., something good happens to the patient) or a "negative" objective outcome measure (i.e., something bad happens to the patient), they can both produce positive and consistent Value Units that can be tracked to determine a combined "total" value.**

Access to Care

Access to care is another objective quality measure that can increase value to a patient by increasing Quality in *the* Value Equation. In order to create a Value Unit scale, a measure of access must first be decided upon. A common unit used to measure patient access in health care is third-next-available appointment (3NA). This shows how far in the future the third next "open spot" is for a patient to have an office visit. A common goal is for a medical provider to have a 3NA of 3 days or less for a regular office visit and 7 days or less for a complete physical examination. This logic would allow us to create an Access to Care Value Unit scale.

Our fictitious example will involve access to care at the orthopedic department. Data is being recorded expressed as third-next-available appointment for access to the orthopedic department (an objective quality measure). A Value Unit scale such as this could be created to convert 3NA data into Value Units:

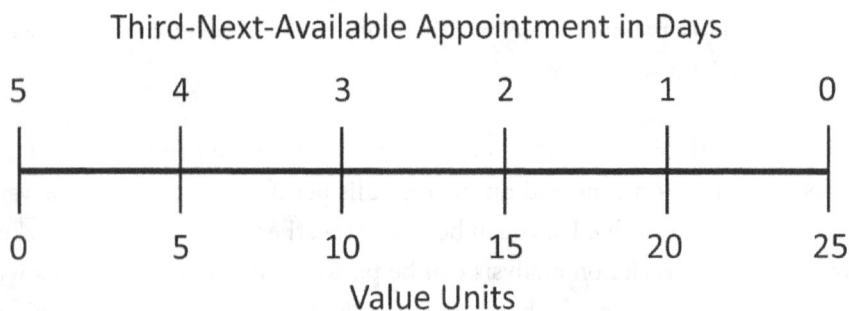

Third-Next-Available Appointment in Days

5	4	3	2	1	0

0	5	10	15	20	25

Value Units

The orthopedic department has set a goal to provide an initial consultation with the third-next-available appointment being on average within 3 days or fewer. If a patient needs to wait five days or more no value is assigned. **Note that this is an example of a "backward" Value Unit scale that measures a "positive" effect for a patient. The shorter the wait time, the greater the value created.**

Appropriateness

Appropriateness increases value by increasing Quality in *the* Value Equation. Appropriateness means measuring whether a service or procedure should have been done in the first place or if it was "appropriately" accurate. If a procedure or service is appropriate for the patient, then it holds value. If a procedure or service is inappropriate, it does not hold value. Value Unit scales converting appropriateness data to Value Units are not much different than other scales except that the logic behind the scales may be simple or quite complicated. For complicated subjects, many "content experts" may be needed to determine what is appropriate and what is not. A more complex example involves looking at CT angiograms to test for heart disease in patients. One section in a cardiology journal shows that it is inappropriate to order this radiology study if a stress test shows moderate to severe ischemia. It is appropriate to order this test if the stress test was equivocal or uninterpretable in certain types of patients. (See "Appropriateness Criteria for Cardiac Computed Tomography and Cardiac Magnetic Resonance Imaging," *Journal of the American College of Cardiology* 48, no. 7 [2006].)

A Value Unit scale could be constructed as such:

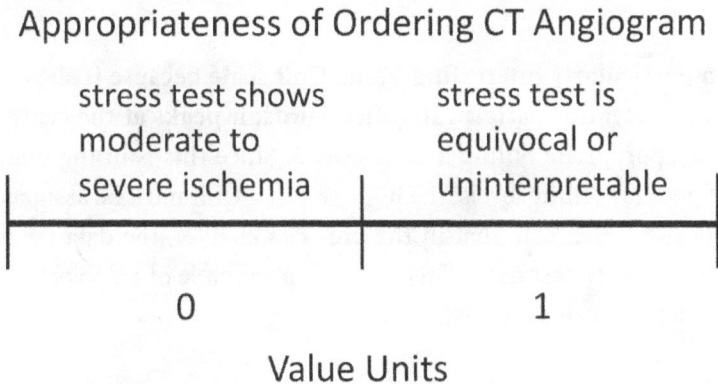

Appropriateness of Ordering CT Angiogram

stress test shows moderate to severe ischemia	stress test is equivocal or uninterpretable
0	1

Value Units

This type of scale is a "range" Value Unit scale as the objective measures can vary but the Value Units assigned are a whole number. **Note that the variance**

in the objective scale this time is *not numbers* (as was the case with the Rogers' adoption curve) but rather a range of possible clinical interpretations ("moderate to severe" and "equivocal or uninterpretable").

Recall from chapter 8 that one of the Value Unit scales determined "appropriate" billing for office visits related to uncomplicated urinary tract infections (they should all be level 3 visits). This Value Unit scale can be retitled and modified to read as such:

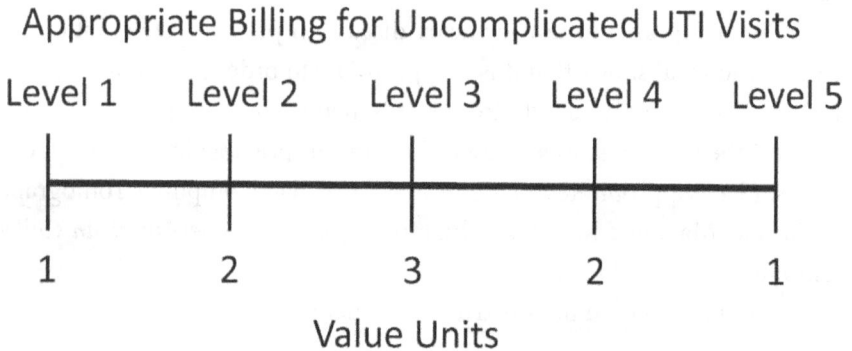

Appropriate Billing for Uncomplicated UTI Visits

Level 1	Level 2	Level 3	Level 4	Level 5
1	2	3	2	1

Value Units

This is a particularly interesting Value Unit scale because it shows a "crescendo-decrescendo" pattern. In other words, it peaks at the center of the scale. The appropriate billing level is level 3. Since this is in the middle of a group of possible billing levels, the highest Value Unit must be assigned to the middle of the scale. Note that in the previous chapter, the data being interpreted was actually cost data. This showed an example of an objective *quality* measure that was using *cost* data!

Medical Record Quality
Improving the quality of a patient's medical record increases value via *the* Value Equation. A chart that has the correct diagnoses, chronic diseases,

allergies, and so forth makes it easier for health care providers to suggest services, manage comorbid diseases, and avoid mistakes. Value Unit scales can be set based on highly specific chart-review criteria (such as all congestive heart failure patients should have CHF written in the problems list of the chart) or basic "field" criteria (such as every patient should at least have something written in the allergy "field"). An example Value Unit scale may look at the percentage of charts that have some data in every clinical field (i.e., allergies, past medical history, past surgical history, family history, social history, etc.):

Percentage of Medical Charts with Data in All Fields

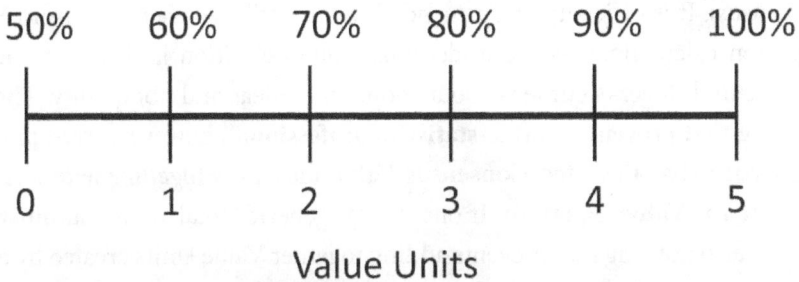

50%	60%	70%	80%	90%	100%

0	1	2	3	4	5

Value Units

The more complete a medical chart is, the higher the value. This example is a simple "forward" Value Unit scale.

Value Unit Scales for Quality and Cost Objective Data Value Calculations

As illustrated in the prior sections, a single cost Value Unit scale can usually be created for a project unless breaking down specific cost elements is truly required. Several quality Value Unit scales may need to be created for a project. Once the Value Unit scales and the logic behind them have been decided upon, they simply must be held constant throughout the project. If all the data is objective, then it can be fairly easily converted to Value Units and calculations performed. The Tier 3 example in chapter 8 illustrates this concept clearly.

Subjective and Objective Value Calculations

All the lessons learned up to this point help make value calculations with subjective and objective data possible. Value Unit scales are, of course, needed. A key question, however, must first be answered:

When can you combine subjective/objective data and when can you not combine subjective/objective data?

If you are not measuring value via *the* Value Equation, then you do not need to combine anything. Consensus Value measures, for example, are independent of *the* Value Equation and are reported without combining any objective data. Recall that Consensus Value measures use a different definition of value (value = consensus). It is officially recommended to keep this data separate from Value Equation calculations as the underlying value definition is different and the logic behind Rogers's curve is about adoption of ideas and not quality. **There is nothing that prevents a value-statistics professional, however, from presenting separately-calculated Consensus Value measures *together with* analyses that use *the* Value Equation.** If one desires generic "total value" summations, there is also nothing that prevents adding together Value Units created by either method. It should be pointed out to an audience, however, that the summation is a combination of Value Units derived from Consensus Value measures and Value Formula–derived measures (dependent on the logic of *the* Value Equation).

Where creation of Value Unit scales is at the most complex level is when Value is being measured via *the* Value Equation and both subjective and objective data are going to be analyzed.

As an example, let us consider an orthopedic "bundle" involving several objective and a subjective data sources that are being measured to look at a more "complete" picture of a service/procedure. Data is being collected for the following:

1) Access to care at the orthopedic department (objective quality measure)(q1)
2) Number of patients discharged on time per day (objective quality measure)(q2)

3) Number of days a patient has moderate-severe pain following hip surgery (subjective quality measure)(q3)
4) Total cost to the patient from initial patient visit to discharge from hospital (objective cost measure)(c1)

The only new information to be introduced here is the total cost of care. If the total cost of care for hip replacement ranged from $20,000–$60,000, a cost Value Unit scale could be created:

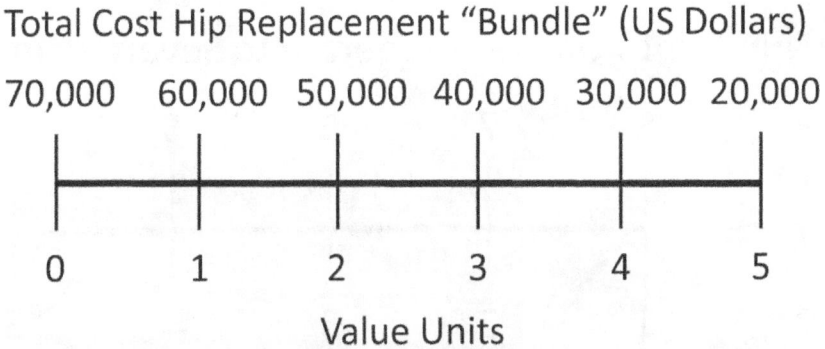

Total Cost Hip Replacement "Bundle" (US Dollars)

70,000   60,000   50,000   40,000   30,000   20,000

0   1   2   3   4   5

Value Units

Note that this is a "backward" scale. The less expensive the service is to a patient, the higher the Value Units assigned. The difficulty does not lie in the creation of Value Unit scales. The other scales involved should look familiar at this point:

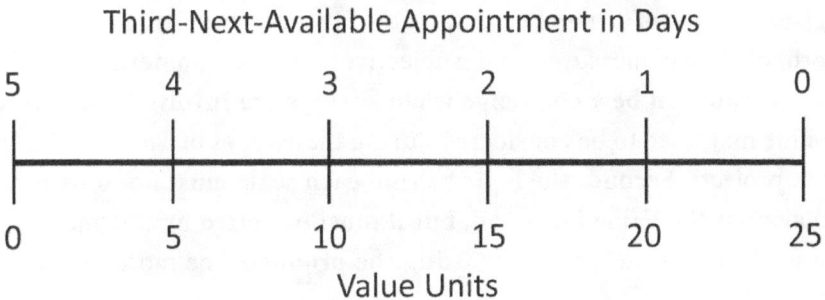

Third-Next-Available Appointment in Days

5   4   3   2   1   0

0   5   10   15   20   25

Value Units

Number of Patients Being Discharged on Time per Day

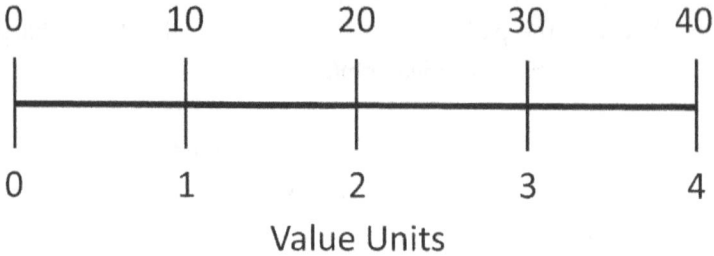

0	10	20	30	40

0	1	2	3	4

Value Units

Number of Days in Moderate to Severe Pain

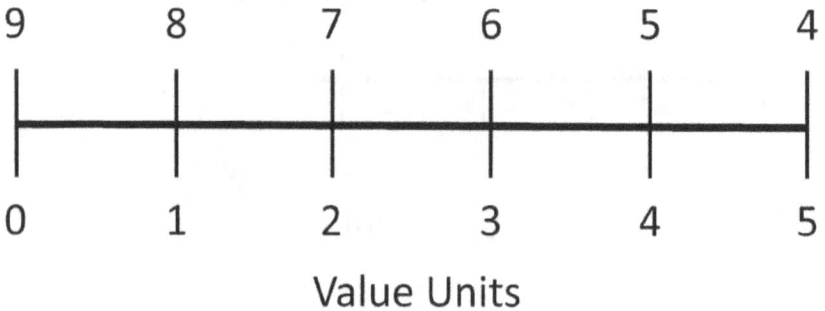

9	8	7	6	5	4

0	1	2	3	4	5

Value Units

The complexity is due to two important logistical points. **First, in a new value-statistics project, the logic for all four of these data sources would need to be created and the resultant data managed simultaneously for a given period of time.** The data is also coming from different sources (both objective measures and subjective surveys). **Sometimes getting _enough_ data can be a challenge when surveys are involved.** As such the n-value may need to be considered during these types of Tier 3* value creation projects. **Second, the logic behind each scale must not only be vetted against _the_ Value Equation, but it must be vetted by the people who are performing the service or using the product.** The more quality and cost measures being analyzed, the higher the chance that changes to the logic behind a Value Unit scale may be modified. At any point along the way, the "content experts" who help value-statistics professionals create the logic behind Value Unit scales may change their minds. It is not the value-statistics professional's role to decide if 4 days of postoperative pain is considered good and 8 days of postoperative days of pain is considered bad. It is the job of the value-statistics professional to reset the Value Unit scale as many times as needed to incorporate the very best logic possible behind the scale. (As mentioned earlier, clinical variation reduction is one method for efficiently creating the clinical standards that often provide the logic needed to set a Value Unit scale). Managing potential changes to multiple Value Unit scales can be challenging. The value calculations based on these Value Unit scales are discussed in the next chapter.

The concept of value measure "bundles" is worth emphasizing. The value assigned to objective outcomes measures such as "number of patients discharged on time per day" can be combined with objective access-to-care measures such as "office visit 3NA" to generate a very basic Value Unit measure that looks at the total value present in both discharge timeliness and follow-up access to care. At the simplest level, these combined Value Units can be tracked over time to see if there is any notable decrease in value from this outcomes-access objective measure (a simple "bundle"). The Value Unit scales and the logic behind them must remain constant. If a subjective quality measure such as the patient reported outcome "number of days in moderate-severe pain" following hip surgery is converted to Value Units, this can also be added to the first two objective measures (creating an outcomes-access-PRO "bundle"), but the Value Unit scale and the logic behind it must remain constant. Finally, the objective cost measure can be placed visually in the denominator to complete the "bundle" measure (outcomes-access-PRO/Cost). While Cost was placed in the denominator to show its corresponding place in *the* Value Equation logic, this is, again, not for performing mathematics.

The only mistake you should never make:

Remember that *the* Value Equation is a *vetting* equation, and not really a mathematical equation. It is acceptable to show where the variables go according to *the* Value Equation:

$$V = \frac{Q}{Cost}$$

$$V = \frac{q1+q2+q3}{c1+c2+c3}$$

If Value Units are placed into this equation, however, the resulting calculations will not make any sense. Since the Value Unit scales are designed to convert cost data into positive Value Units, the scale itself is "removing the math" from the results. In other words, if you put more and more positive Value Units into the denominator of *the* Value Equation, you will shrink or decrease the calculated value rather than increase it. So don't make that mistake!

Value Unit scales keep the logic of *the* Value Equation the same but simplify the mathematics to the previously demonstrated versions:

$$\uparrow V = \uparrow Q + \downarrow C$$

and

$$\Delta V = \Delta Q + \Delta C$$

Also, trying to create Value Unit scales for cost data that shows fractions in order to use *the* Value Equation for direct calculations will only create unneeded complexity and difficulties. As the first paragraph of this chapter stated, Value Units are designed to make the mathematics easier and the interpretation of the data more accurate.

The more complex Value Formulas become, the greater the challenge to understand if value continues to be created, if is it growing or shrinking in a concerning way, and what the source of a significant rise or fall may be. Yet a few more skills are needed to efficiently monitor the sustainability and growth of value creation.

For a practical approach to organizing Value Unit scales, see "The Five Golden Steps of Value Unit Scale Creation" in chapter 11.

10

VALUE SUSTAINABILITY AND IMPROVEMENT—MEASURING VALUE AND ADDRESSING TOTAL COST OF CARE

"We keep moving forward, opening new doors, and doing new things, because we're curious and curiosity keeps leading us down new paths."—Walt Disney

After being able to predict if value will be created using *the* Value Equation, measure for sure that it is being created using Value Formulas and converting the value measures to Value Units (to ease calculations and understanding); the next step is to sustain successful value improvement projects. This involves adding the element of rolling time to previous analytics. It also involves introducing the concept of variation reduction. **Incorporating these two elements allows value-statistics professionals to begin measuring quality and total cost of care as value.** It should be emphasized that although "total cost of care" has grabbed headlines recently, it is still just a cost measure (albeit a compound measure) and only part of the thought process involved in more comprehensive value calculations.

Variation reduction is a branch of statistical analytics that searches for variations in data that actually signify an important change. Displaying data in control charts (also known as XMR or Shewhart charts) is a common way to determine if data is displaying "common cause variation" (within expected controls) or "special cause variation" (not within expected controls). (Consider reading *Understanding Variation—The Key to Managing Chaos* by Donald Wheeler if a quick review of variation statistics is needed.)

Since *the* Value Equation and subjective-objective data conversion to Value Units has been adequately introduced, the next major hurdle in value measurement is sustainability and improvement. When looking at the Value Units determined from any Value Unit scale individually, a control chart can be constructed to determine if the value creation from that objective or subjective measure is still in control. If the Value Units go over the upper control limit (UCL), then unexpectedly more value than usual was created. If the Value Units fall under the lower control limit (LCL), then unexpectedly less value than usual was created. If the Value Units stay between the control limits (CLs), then the value creation is at the current "normal state" for the service or product. While there are additional rules that determine when a "trend" is important, this chapter will not expand upon that concept.

Measuring Value Creation from Quality

Let us revisit our example of access to care at the orthopedic department. Data being recorded is expressed as third-next-available appointment for access to the orthopedic department (an objective quality measure). A Value Unit scale was created to convert this raw data into Value Units.

Third-Next-Available Appointment in Days

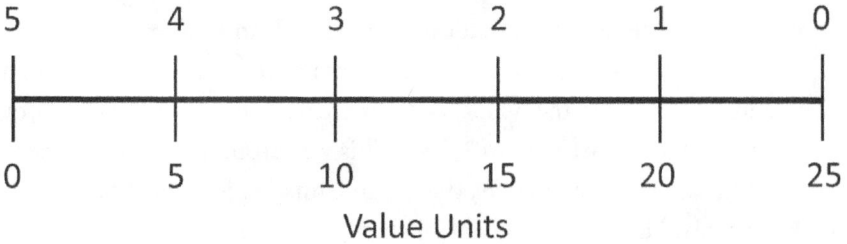

5	4	3	2	1	0

0	5	10	15	20	25

Value Units

The orthopedic department has set a goal to provide an initial consultation with the third-next-available appointment being on average within 3 days or fewer. When converted to Value Units, this access-to-care objective measure would result in 10 Value Units or greater. The providers and staff have tried a few different strategies to improve access (one around February 16 and another around April 20) and the resultant value measure. They would like to know how much value they are creating and if either of their efforts helped them reach their goal.

The access-to-care objective data in Value Units can be plotted over time as a control chart (the moving range chart is not included for simplification):

Value Generated by Access to Care

Orthopedic Department January 2011–May 2011

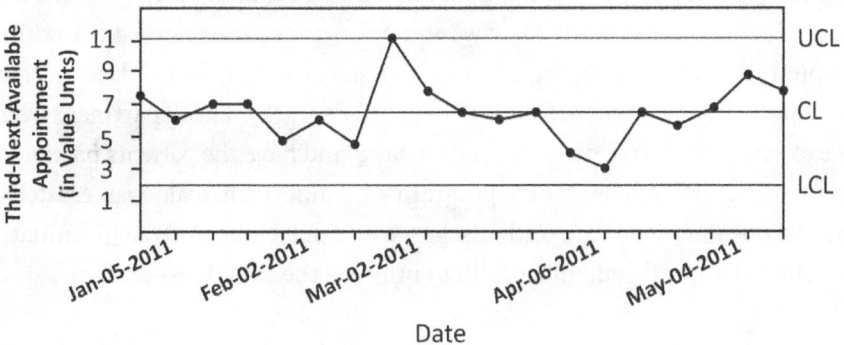

The control chart shows that the average value created for this time period was between 6 and 7 Value Units (the line between the oscillating data points). The Value Unit scale shows us that this corresponds to an average third-next-available appointment of 3–4 days, which does not meet the department goal. At the end of February, the Value Units increased to over 10, which would correspond to a 3NA earlier than 3 days. This was around the time of the first strategic initiative. Unfortunately, the Value Units fell just short of exceeding the upper control limit for this control chart. This means that this increase is still considered common cause variation and cannot be attributed to the strategic initiative. This is supported by the following data, which does not show the 3NA Value Units staying above the average. The second strategic initiative also did not appear to increase the value in any way that could not be attributed to random common cause variation.

In this case, the control chart helps answer questions about sustainability and attempts to increase value creation. Although the strategic initiatives failed to create a higher level of value through access to care, the department can still be reassured that they are sustaining value at the current level. At no time did the Value Units dip below the lower control limit, so at least the strategic initiatives did not have a negative impact. The department can regroup and consider a different approach.

Let us review our example of hospital discharges related to the orthopedic department.

The orthopedic department has data related to discharge times from the hospital following hip surgery. They want to measure value created due to timely hospital discharges. Keeping all standard safety measures in place, patients were discharged anywhere from 3–7 days after surgery. The department would like to safely discharge patients around day 3 and have the patients participate in an outpatient rehabilitation program. A Value Unit scale was created to convert postoperative days until discharge to Value Units. A strategic initiative was started around September 2010 to improve the timeliness of discharges.

The Value Unit scale is as follows:

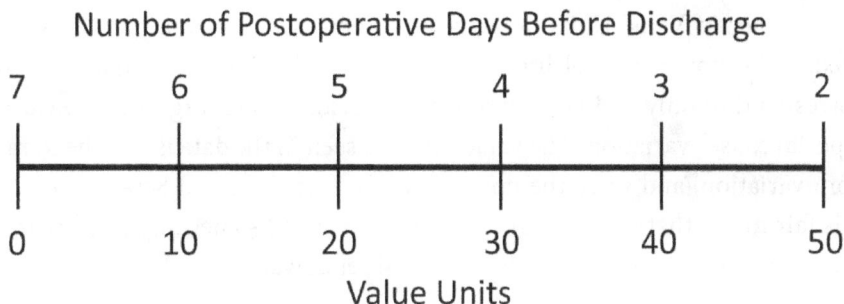

Number of Postoperative Days Before Discharge

7	6	5	4	3	2

0	10	20	30	40	50

Value Units

The orthopedic department wants to know if the value created by timely discharges has increased and if the strategic initiative contributed to the increased value creation.

The "timely discharge" objective data in Value Units can be plotted over time as a control chart (the moving range chart is not included for simplification):

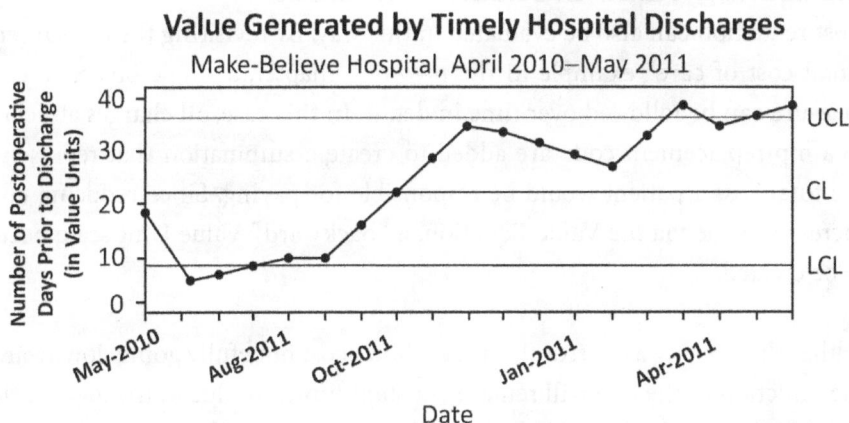

Value Generated by Timely Hospital Discharges
Make-Believe Hospital, April 2010–May 2011

Although the average Value Units for the time displayed on the control chart are around 25 (corresponding to 4–5 postoperative days before discharge), there is a clear trend present. Since the strategic initiative in September 2010, the number of Value Units did appear to increase. Two data points also exceeded the upper control limit (UCL). Those Value Units (around 35–40) correspond to only 3–4 postoperative days prior to discharge and are clearly "special cause" variation. The value increase seen in the data is not due to random variation, and since the upward climb started around September 2010, it is fair to say that the strategic initiative likely had something to do with it. Over time, the average Value Unit line will set upward.

It should be noted that Value Unit control charts always show value creation going upward and value loss heading downward. This consistent "up is good" and "down is bad" makes for straightforward analyses. Ease of interpretation is possible, again, because of the conversion of all data into Value Units. Value control charts illustrate and reinforce the principle that the purpose of Value Units is to make calculations and interpretations easier.

Measuring Value Creation from Cost

Cost reduction can also be evaluated in this way. By revisiting the hip surgery "total cost of care" example in the previous chapter, a single objective cost measure can be followed over time in detail. In this case, all charges attached to a hip replacement code are added to create a summation that represents the total cost a patient would be responsible for paying. Since reducing cost increases value via *the* Value Equation, a "backward" Value Unit scale needs to be created.

Rather than seeing a control chart that shows cost hopefully going downward, the direction of the line will remain constant (upward) due to the logic of the Value Unit scale. In the case of control charts, the goal is always to increase the data points above the upper control limit (UCL) showing special cause value creation.

The following shows the Value Unit scale for total cost hip replacement:

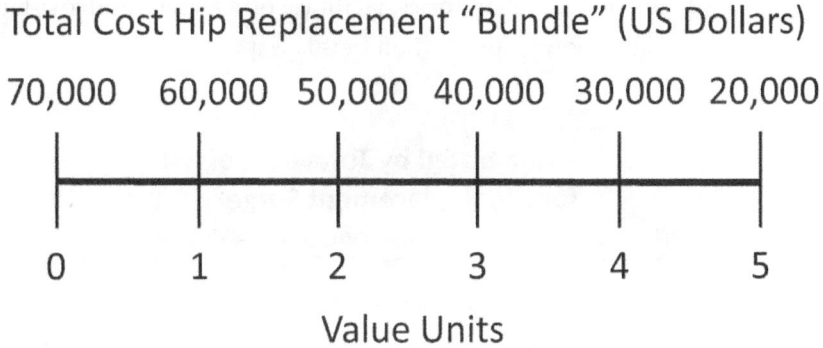

Total Cost Hip Replacement "Bundle" (US Dollars)

70,000	60,000	50,000	40,000	30,000	20,000

0	1	2	3	4	5

Value Units

If the goal was to get the total cost of care for hip replacement surgeries down to $40,000, a control chart such as this would be useful:

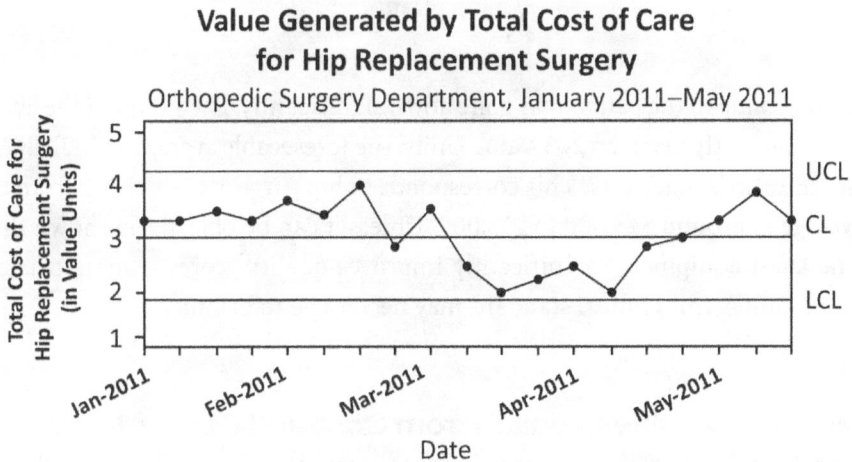

**Value Generated by Total Cost of Care
for Hip Replacement Surgery**
Orthopedic Surgery Department, January 2011–May 2011

In this example, the average Value Units score is about 3, which corresponds to $40,000. Also, the cost fluctuates within the control limits, so it can be predicted that the average cost would remain about the same under current conditions.

Alternatively, if a clinical standard by the local orthopedic surgeons was created around March 2011 that involved utilizing "the latest equipment" in addition to all of the previous laboratories, facilities, office visits, and assistants, a control chart might show value creation in this way:

Value Generated by Total Cost of Care for Hip Replacement Surgery

Orthopedic Surgery Department, January 2011–May 2011

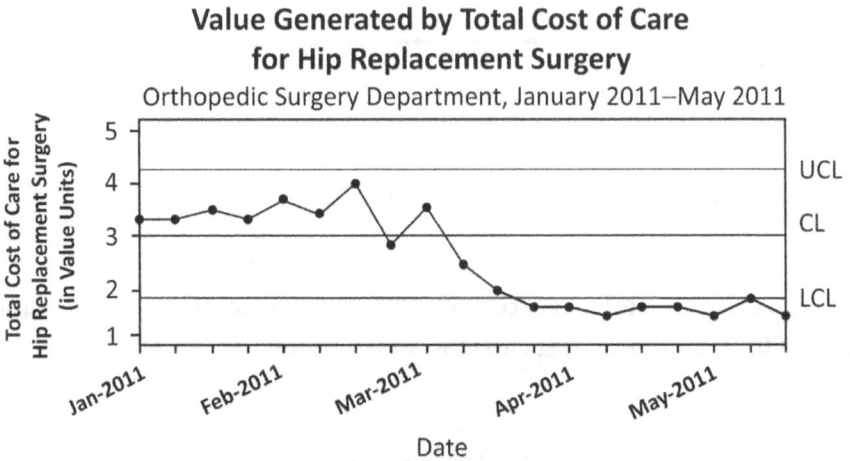

Clearly value to the patient has gone down significantly. Even though the average is currently between 2–3 Value Units, the foreseeable average will likely be closer to 1.5 Value Units. This corresponds to hip surgery costs rising from an average of around $45,000 to $55,000. Unless it can be objectively shown that "the latest equipment" significantly improves quality scores (and associated Value Units), this clinical standard may need to be reformulated.

Measuring Value Creation from Cost and Quality Together

Now that this chapter has shown individual cost and quality examples, it will continue to demonstrate the true usefulness of Value Units by showing how **compound value measures composed of both quality and cost components can be effectively measured and efficiently interpreted**. When quality and cost values measures are to be analyzed together, the result is called a **Compound Value**

measure. The cost and quality elements are called **Component Value measures**. This terminology is carried forward during analyses. A control chart displaying cost data, for example, could be called a *Component* Value control chart.

The following will discuss a few rules that are unique to compound value measure calculations.

These are the "rules of thumb" when it comes to compound value measures:

1) Try to set all quality and cost Value Unit scales to show single digit Value Units[†] (preferably 0–5 or 0–10).

2) Try to predict the maximum amount of cost that can be saved for objective cost measures, then set the Value Unit scale accordingly (although 1% of the maximum predicted cost savings is the minimum Value Unit recommended, it should commonly be set higher; a cost variation graph can also be used†).

3) Remember that quality measures can have a maximum, so consider drawing a "ceiling line" on control charts to reflect this value and plan quality Value Unit scales accordingly.

4) Always have all *Component* Value control charts visible when assessing a *Compound* Value control chart and *Subcomponent* Value control charts visible when assessing *Component* Value charts.

[†]This rule is part of the Five Golden Steps of Value Unit Scale Creation, detailed in chapter 11.

Definition of Value #18

Component Value = all cost components (or quality components) expressed as Value Units summed for the purpose of creating a Compound Value calculation

(Based on the vetting Value Equation, Component Values can be thought of as synonymous with the "big Q" and "big C" elements; while the subcomponents would relate to the "little q" and "little c" elements)

Definition of Value #19

Compound Value = a total value summation combining Cost Component Value and Quality Component Value

Rule #1 was demonstrated in the "hip replacement total cost of care" example. When individually looking at cost or quality value creation, the Value Unit scale range (i.e., 1–5 or 5–50) does not make as much difference as long as it is held constant. When multiple Value Unit sources are combined, however, a scale showing large numbers will radically shift the *Compound* Value control chart. While this does not technically cause errors (a new average and control limits can always be determined), it can be distracting when presenting the data to others. **If a Value Unit scale of 1–5 or 0–5 can realistically be assigned to all quality and cost value measures, the resulting *Compound* Value control chart will appear "more stable."**

Rule #2 was introduced in chapter 9. It is always easier to sum all costs into a single measure and set the Value Scale accordingly. Sometimes, however, knowing which cost elements are contributing more can be important. In this circumstance all cost value measures ("little c" components) must have their own Value Unit scales and control charts. The summation of all "little c" cost value measures will then result in the "big C" Cost value measure and *Component* Value control chart.

Here is an example of creating a Compound Value measure.
This example has three parts. Here is Part 1:
An organization wants to measure value creation for hip surgeries using a Tier 3* value creation model. The cost value measure elements will be as follows (all objective cost measures):

1) Average laboratory costs per patient
2) Average office visit costs per patient
3) Average radiology study costs per patient
4) Average surgery costs per patient

In this case it is already known that these cost measures will become a Component Value measure (all cost components combined). As such, the Value Unit scales for each value measure will follow rule #2. The raw data shows that average laboratory costs ranged from $80–$250. The office visit costs ranged from $100–$350. The radiology study costs ranged from $500–$2,500. The average surgery costs ranged from $5,000–$25,000. While the organization may want to set more aggressive targets, basic Value Unit scales can already be set:

Average Radiology Study Cost per Patient (US Dollars)

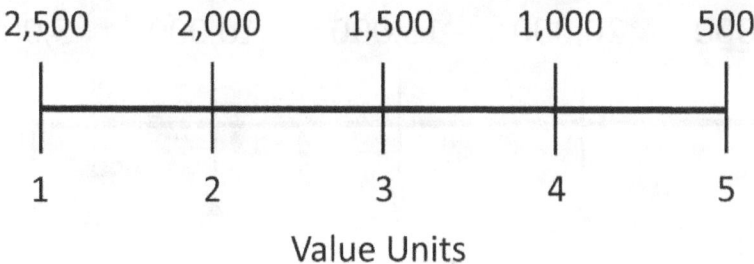

2,500	2,000	1,500	1,000	500
1	2	3	4	5

Value Units

Average Office Visit Cost per Patient (US Dollars)

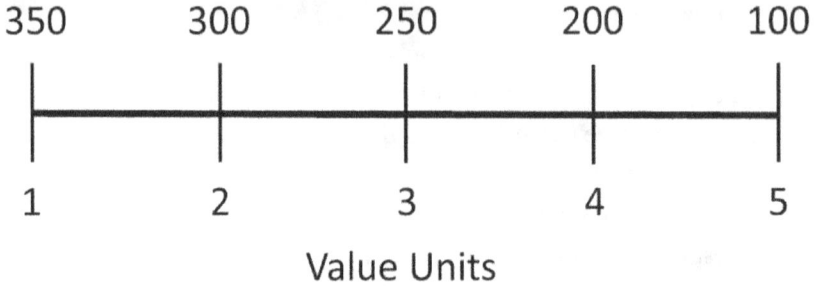

350	300	250	200	100
1	2	3	4	5

Value Units

Average Surgery Cost per Patient (US Dollars)

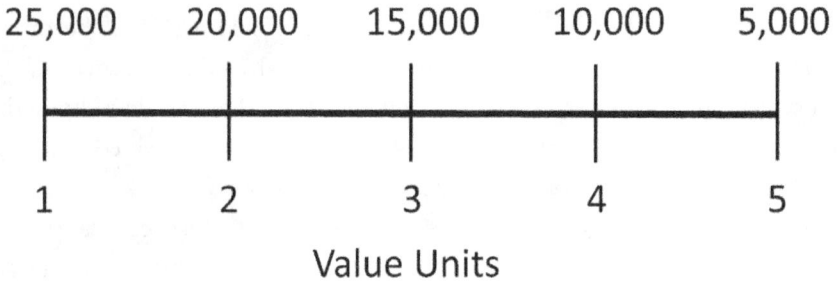

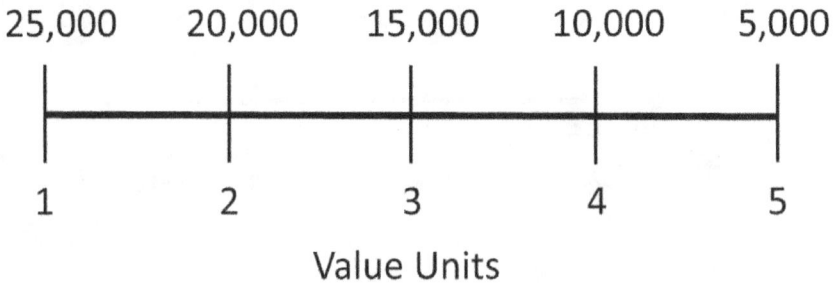

25,000	20,000	15,000	10,000	5,000
1	2	3	4	5

Value Units

Average Surgery Cost per Patient (US Dollars)

25,000	20,000	15,000	10,000	5,000
1	2	3	4	5

Value Units

Note that while the objective cost measures (upper part of the scale) vary considerably, the Value Unit scales are all single digits and consistent. Rule #2 also reminds us that in theory costs could go below the numbers shown on right side of the scale. If this happened unexpectedly, the Value Unit scales would need to be adjusted accordingly. Objective cost data can now be converted to Value Units and tracked over time. Control charts can be created for each objective cost measure and Value Unit scale:

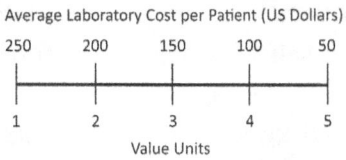

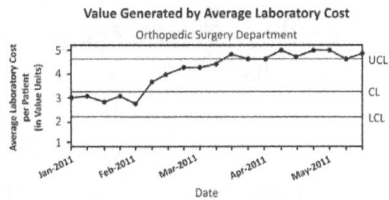

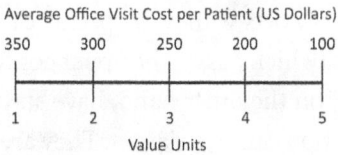

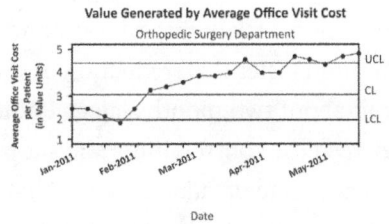

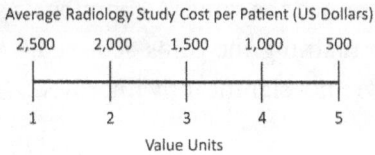

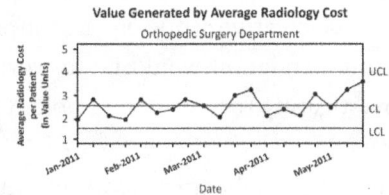

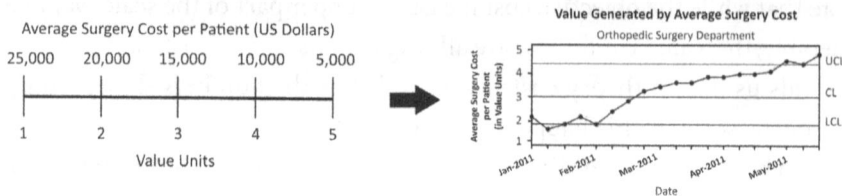

Average Surgery Cost per Patient (US Dollars)

25,000   20,000   15,000   10,000   5,000

1   2   3   4   5

Value Units

Value Generated by Average Surgery Cost
Orthopedic Surgery Department

A great deal of information can be derived from this initial presentation of data. Flexibility, however, is still present and remains the strength of this method. If one does not desire average charges per patient, for example, the raw total costs for each category could be used. Once this chain of analysis is structured, the data used and the Value Unit scale logic can always be modified as the needs of an organization evolve. Nevertheless, quickly looking at these control charts created from the logic of the Value Unit scales shows us that value is being created. Value has increased over time to the level of special cause variation for cost reduction in laboratory costs, office visit costs, and surgery costs. Reduction of laboratory costs and office visits costs achieved special cause variation faster than reduction of surgery costs (which passes the upper control limit about two months later). Radiology cost, on the other hand, have stayed between the control limits and show only common cause variation. They are at a steady state of value creation that has neither improved or worsened. When it comes to cost reduction for this project, a value-statistics professional can report that three cost reduction measures have shown notable improvement in value creation while one measure has remained the same. A commonsense recommendation would be to work on maintaining the gains achieved and investigating further why radiology costs were not significantly improved.

Each of the subcomponents, or "little c" components, can be a project of its own and monitored in this way. As these subcomponents are part of a Tier 3* project, in this case one additional step is needed. The subcomponents need to be combined to create a **Cost Component Value** analysis. In this case, all the Value Units for each data collection point (the dots on the control charts) are added together to create a "total value" from cost reduction. The control chart y-axis needs to be changed to range from 4–20 as the maximum Value Units that can be achieved by the logic of these *four* Value Unit scales is 20 and the minimum is 4. **It is now clear why setting consistent and simple Value Unit scales is important for Tier 3 projects.** All Value Unit scales for subcomponents will ultimately affect the Component Value control chart.

The information gained from looking at a Cost Component Value control chart is different than the individual subcomponent control charts:

Component Value Generated by Cost Reduction

Orthopedic Surgery Department

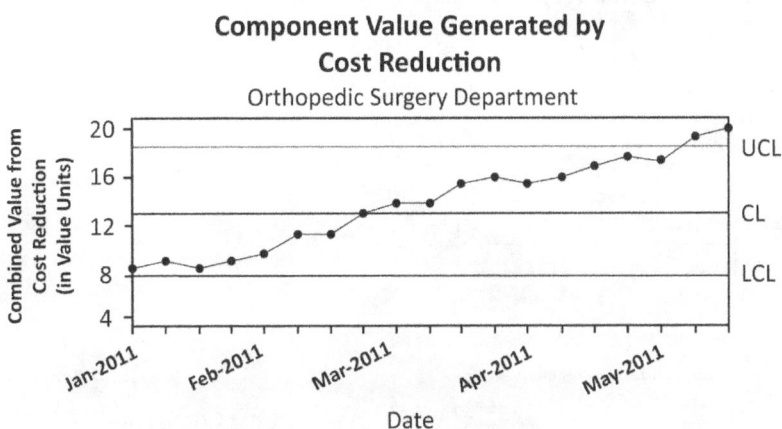

When the combined cost Value Units are combined and analyzed, a steady trend of value creation is observed. The line does not cross the upper control limit until the very end of time frame, however. While it is clear that cost reduction has contributed to value creation, in this case it is more difficult to understand why as this represents a "bundle" measure. By combining multiple objective cost measures, an overall picture of value creation has been achieved but at the expense of understanding what contributed the most.

Recall that Rule #4 states that a value-statistics professional should have all *Subcomponent* Value control charts visible when assessing a *Component* Value control chart. This is because the "little c" subcomponents in this case explain the why whereas the "big C" component demonstrates if the "bundle" effort was successful as a whole or not.

Examining the subcomponent control charts alongside the Cost Component Value control chart provides a more complete understanding of this part 1 analysis. The cost reduction "bundle" effort was successful according to the Cost Component Value control chart. The success was due to cost reduction in laboratory costs, office visits, and surgery costs according to the subcomponent control charts. The success was not achieved until the end of this time frame because the radiology costs did not decrease enough to raise value above the upper control limit (stalling value creation) and the surgical costs only achieved special cause variation at the very end (delaying cumulative value creation).

"Little c"
Subcomponents

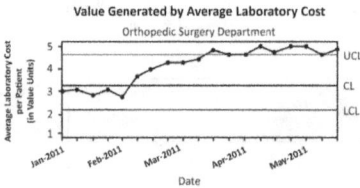

c1

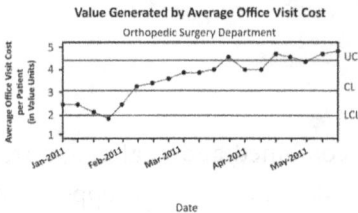

c2

"Big C"
Cost Component Value

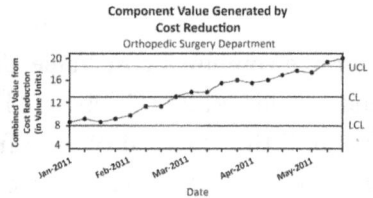

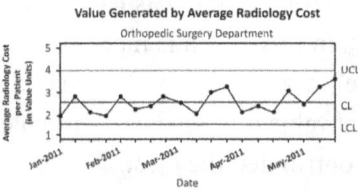

c3

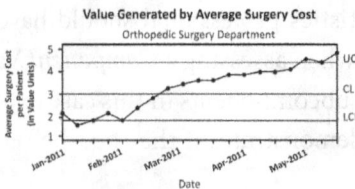

c4

Part 1 of this Tier 3* analysis is now complete. It shows the creation of a Cost Component Value analysis and the subcomponents. This can also be thought of as a Cost "bundle."

Here is part 2:

The next step is to produce a similar analysis on desired Quality components around hip replacement surgery. The quality value measure elements will be as follows:

1) Office visit access, third-next-available appointment (objective quality measure—access to care)
2) Days until discharge following surgery (objective quality measure—outcome)
3) Days in moderate to severe pain after surgery (subjective quality measure—patient reported outcome)
4) Percentage of patients that develop DVT (deep vein thrombosis) or PE (pulmonary embolism) following surgery (objective quality measure—outcome)

Value Unit scales will be created for each of these data sources using some content-expert input to set the scales as accurately as possible. The orthopedic department considers good patient access (measured in third-next-available appointment) to be within 5 days. The surgeons feel that discharging a patient from the hospital within 3 days to begin outpatient therapy is ideal. A group of orthopedists, nurses, and patients decided that having a patient out of severe pain, off of prescription medications, within 10 days would be excellent and that being on prescription pain medications for longer than 25 days would be less desirable. As all patients receive prophylactic anticoagulation, the surgeons would be disappointed if the DVT or PE percentage was above 20% based on current evidence-based medicine. The Value Units scales can now be set:

Office Visit Access (Third-Next-Available Appointment)

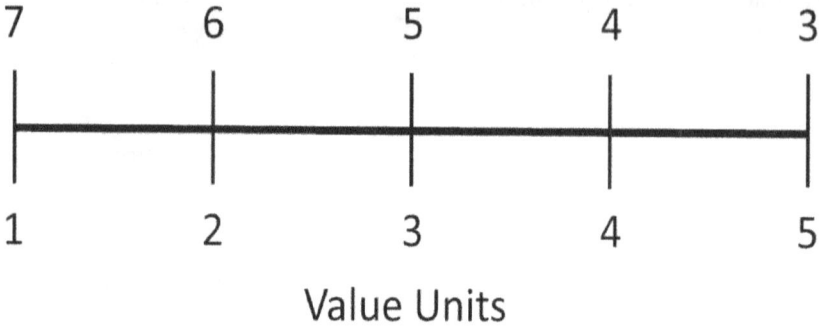

7	6	5	4	3
1	2	3	4	5

Value Units

Postoperative Days Until Discharge

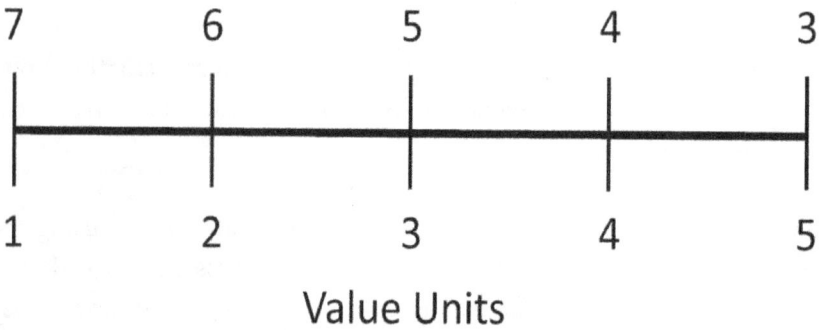

7	6	5	4	3
1	2	3	4	5

Value Units

Postoperative Days in Severe Pain

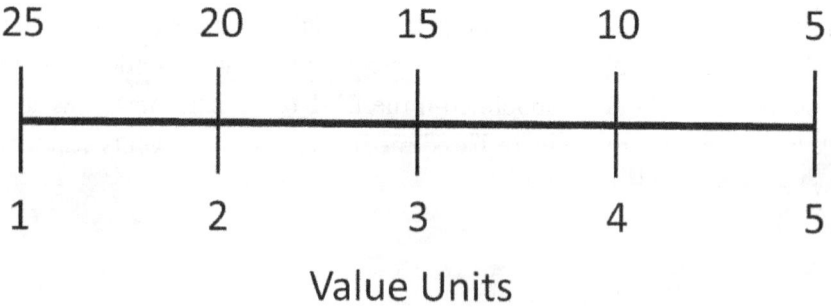

25	20	15	10	5
1	2	3	4	5

Value Units

DVT/PE Percentage Rate in Postoperative Patients

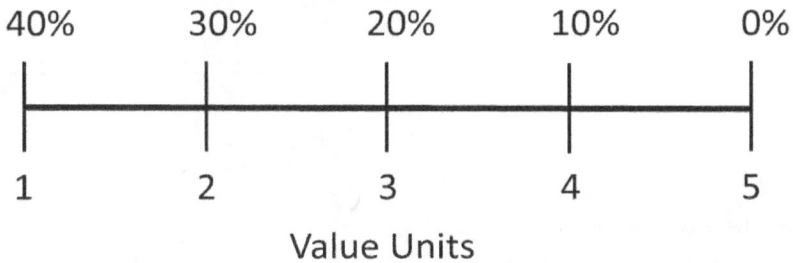

Note again that while the subjective and objective quality measure on the top of the scale can vary, the Value Unit part of the scale is consistent and set to single digits. The subjective and objective quality data can now be converted to Value Units and tracked over time. Control charts can be created for each objective cost measure and Value Unit scale:

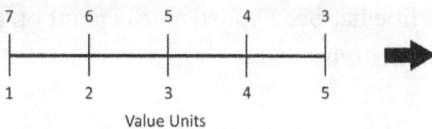

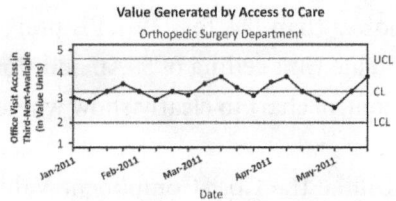

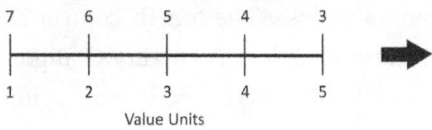

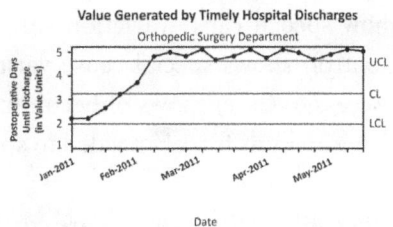

Postoperative Days in Severe Pain

25	20	15	10	5
1	2	3	4	5

Value Units

Value Generated by Postoperative Pain Control
Orthopedic Surgery Department

DVT/PE Percentage Rate in Postoperative Patients

40%	30%	20%	10%	0%
1	2	3	4	5

Value Units

Value Generated by DVT and PE Prevention
Orthopedic Surgery Department

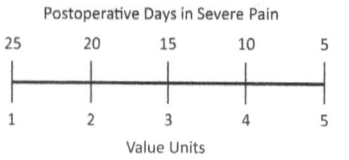

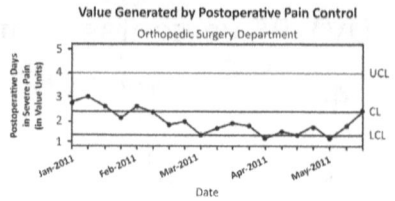

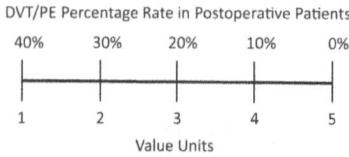

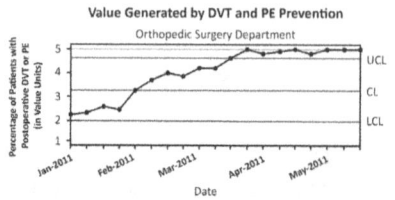

Rule #3 reminds us that some quality subcomponents may have a maximum value. Out of the four examples shown here, only the DVT/PE Value Unit scale and control chart reach a "quality maximum." Since it is not possible to go lower than 0% for DVT/PE prevention, this corresponds with a maximum Value Unit ceiling of 5. An additional line has been added at this point on the control chart to clearly show where the ceiling exists.

Unlike the Cost Component Value analysis, the quality data shown here is a "mixed bag." Two control charts (Timely Discharges, DVT/PE Prevention) show special cause variation value creation. One chart (Postoperative Pain Control) shows special cause variation value loss. The fourth control chart (Access to Care) shows only common cause variation. A Quality Component Value analysis is truly needed to sort out if value was created overall or not.

When all quality elements are combined, the Quality Component Value control chart looks like this:

Component Value Generated by Quality

Orthopedic Surgery Department

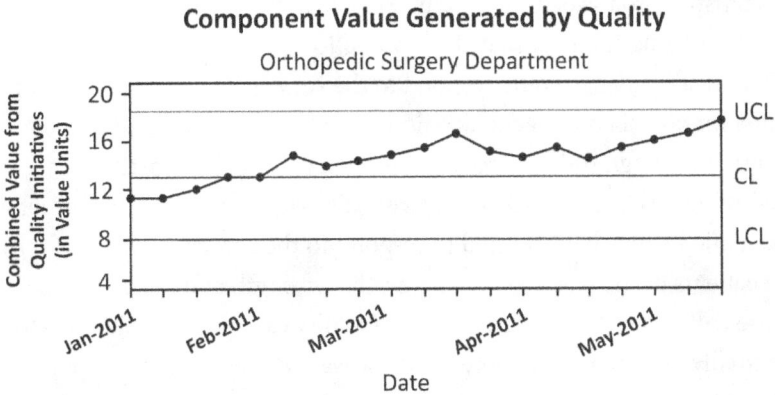

While there is a clear trend toward value creation, the line does not cross the upper control limit. The trend is significant but not as dramatic as the rise above the upper control limit seen with the Cost Component Value control chart. Clearly the value loss observed in the postoperative pain control initiative and the common cause variation seen with the access-to-care initiative have stifled more noticeable value creation for this Quality "bundle."

As was previously mentioned, this Quality Component Value analysis is useful for direction, trend, and a "bundle" perspective. It does not explain why the trend was somewhat positive but not dramatic. It also does not provide guidance as to what quality elements need to be improved.

Following Rule #4 allows for a more detailed understanding of the Quality Component Value analysis and potential strategic decision making. When the subcomponent control charts are placed next to the Quality Component Value control chart, some additional important observations can be made. An apparent slight to the value creation project is that the postoperative pain control seemed to be steadily worsening even though the organization was making a concerted effort to improve this quality measure. **An immediate statistical concern is that this is the only subjective quality outcome measure (patient reported outcome) and may be less reliable data than the three objective quality measures.** A value-statistics professional may want to look at the survey response rate as one assumption being made is that the n-value for all measures is the same. In an ideal world, all patients would respond to the survey, and the n-value (number of patients) for all subcomponents would be the same. Recall the discussion about "strength and magnitude" introduced in chapter 3. All the patients in question needed office visits, hospitalization (with discharge), and DVT/PE prophylaxis. Not all patients may have wanted to respond to the survey, however. If only 50% of the patients participated in the survey, the "strength and magnitude" of the q3 measure will be less. This means that the Quality Component Value control chart may actually be affected in a more favorable way. While these calculations will not be shown here, they should be kept in mind whenever subjective quality outcome measures such as patient reported outcomes are being used.

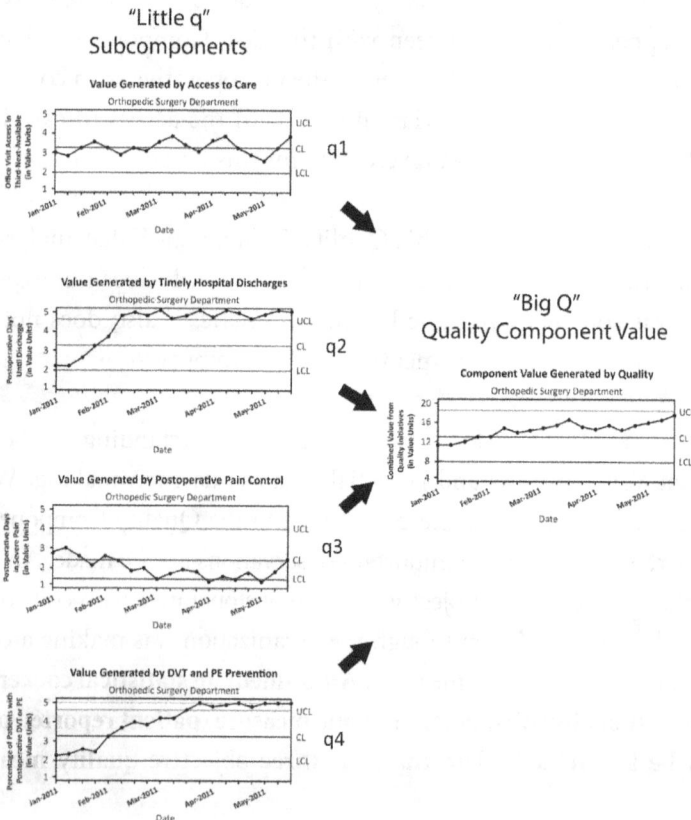

"Little q"
Subcomponents

Value Generated by Access to Care
Orthopedic Surgery Department

q1

Value Generated by Timely Hospital Discharges
Orthopedic Surgery Department

q2

"Big Q"
Quality Component Value

Component Value Generated by Quality
Orthopedic Surgery Department

Value Generated by Postoperative Pain Control
Orthopedic Surgery Department

q3

Value Generated by DVT and PE Prevention
Orthopedic Surgery Department

q4

Part 2 of this Tier 3* analysis is now complete. It shows the creation of a Quality Component Value analysis and the subcomponents. This can also be thought of as a Quality "bundle."

The final step, or part 3, is to create a Compound Value analysis utilizing the Cost Component Value and the Quality Component Value elements. When the Value Units of each Component Value data set are combined, a new Compound Value control chart can be constructed. As there are now 8 different subcomponents represented (c1, c2, c3, c4, q1, q2, q3, q4), the scale on the control chart must be adjusted to range from 8 to 40. **Note that the y-axis of each control chart is simply "added" together to allow for the combined Value Unit scores.**

"Big C"
Cost Component Value

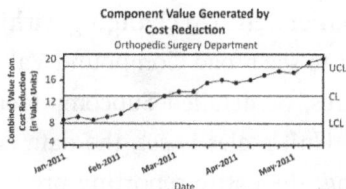

"Total"
Compound Value

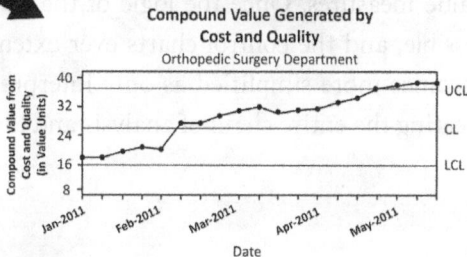

"Big Q"
Quality Component Value

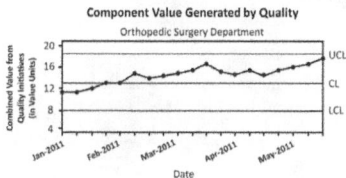

When all elements of value creation are looked at together in the Compound Value control chart, the success of the endeavor is self-evident. Not only is there a consistent trend showing value creation, but the upper control limit actually has been exceeded by the end of this time interval. As Rule #4 reminds us, the Component Value control charts are needed to understand the "Total" Compound Value in more detail. While success was achieved, the cost reduction efforts contributed the most to the success. Even though quality efforts did not generate value as dramatically as the cost reduction component, there clearly was not an overall sacrifice to the quality measures. Quality did not go down as a "bundle" but rather appeared to inch upward.

When data collection is readily available or automated, these interconnected control charts can endlessly "roll forward" and show if value continues to be created and sustained. Value-statistics professionals can look at this set of "living" value measures and interpret them at various levels. **It is not the final compound control chart that is always in question but rather the changing subcomponent charts within the compound control chart. In other words it is sometimes more useful to observe each smaller delta (Δ) changing within the greater delta (Δ).** Organizations may want to see broad Compound Value measures, focused Component Value measures, or detailed Subcomponent Value measures. Once the logic of the Value Unit scales is set, the data accessible, and the control charts ever extending, the entire reporting process becomes more simplified as only interpretation is now needed (rather than creating the entire chain of analysis and logic).

"Little c"
Subcomponents

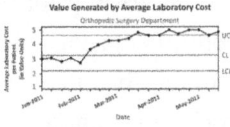 c1

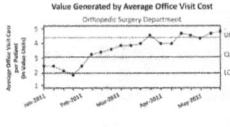 c2

"Big C"
Cost Component Value

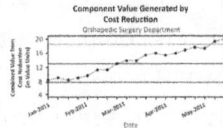

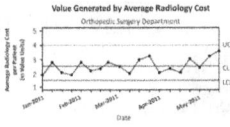 c3

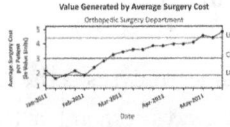 c4

"Total"
Compound Value

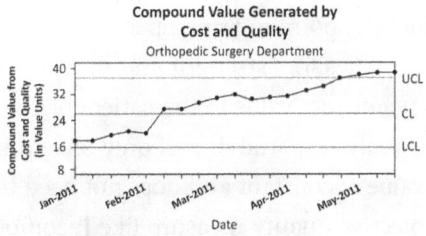

"Little q"
Subcomponents

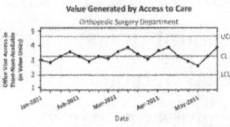 q1

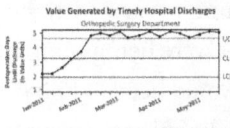 q2

"Big Q"
Quality Component Value

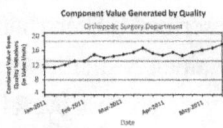

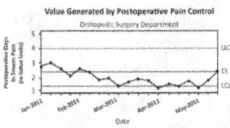 q3

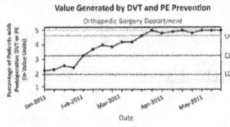 q4

These control charts rise and fall as value is created and lost. Successes and failures can quickly be identified. Strategic planning allows one to prioritize which elements of a value creation plan need to be discontinued, adjusted, or simply sustained. Tier 3 "bundles" can also be increased by adding more quality and cost subcomponents (i.e., c_5, q_5) if an organization deems it necessary.

While this form of value analysis is not necessarily easy to create, it is quite *easy to interpret* once the creation is complete. **Up means value is going up. Down means value is going down.** Each subcomponent measure flows into a component measure, which in turn flows into a compound measure. With the risk of sounding redundant, **the entire point of using Value Unit scales and this methodology is to achieve a resulting value measure that anyone can learn to interpret in a short period of time regardless of expertise**.

The final point to remember when it comes to Tier 3* value analyses is the use of n-values for "strength and magnitude" calculations. Always remember that value means "value to the patient or customer." Value comes from every person the analysis is studying. If only one group of people is being looked at, then the n-value is constant and does not need to be taken into account unless a partial subjective quality measure like incomplete patient reported outcomes is being used (previously discussed in this chapter). However, n-values are particularly important if two groups are being evaluated under the same value statistics logic. For example, if two different orthopedic surgery groups were being compared using the same "bundle" logic described earlier, then we would need to know the number of patients involved (n-value). A smaller orthopedic surgery group that provides the best care may still generate less overall value when compared to a large orthopedic surgery group that provides excellent care. Recall that Value Units derived from subjective data can be multiplied by the n-value to generate "total value" scores that incorporate "strength and magnitude." (Chapter 3 introduces this concept within the context of Consensus Value measurements, but the logic can be used for calculations based on *the* Value Equation as well.)

When multiple groups are being compared using a Tier 3 "bundle" logic, an umbrella term that can be applied to describe the required enormous amount of data analysis is "**mega bundle**."

One purpose of this chapter is primarily to demonstrate the incredible flexibility available when it comes to setting up Value Unit scales. The end of the next chapter presents a more straightforward, practical approach to the creation and utilization of Value Unit scales for typical everyday projects.

11

A PRACTICAL APPROACH—PUTTING IT ALL TOGETHER

"The secret to getting ahead is getting started."—Mark Twain

The main rule for a value-statistics professional will always be to **keep things as simple as possible**. Do not do more than is needed or increase the complexity of an analysis unless it is deemed necessary. *Just because you know how to do it does not mean you should do it.*

This chapter will illustrate how to visually simplify tiered value measures, utilize Value Quotients, and most importantly create Value Unit scales in a practical way (The Five Golden Steps of Value Unit Scale Creation).

Starting Tiered Value Measure Projects

If an organization is smaller and has only one or two people dedicated to value creation projects, then the commonsense, practical approach is to start by defining Tier 1 projects or Consensus Value projects. Take one project of each type from beginning to end and identify where challenges existed. Try to determine the following:

1) Were there any problems choosing a project topic?
2) Were there any problems defining value (setting Consensus Value questions or creating Value Unit scales)?
3) Were there any problems measuring value (getting the data needed)?
4) Were there any problems determining if value was being created fast enough and in a balanced manner (strategic planning)?
5) Were there any problems sustaining value creation or measurement?
6) Can the entire process be repeated in a more organized and efficient way?
7) Who is best suited for completing each part needed to finish a project?
8) Is the team ready for a higher tier project?

There is nothing more satisfying than completing a project and demonstrating positive value creation. As such, organizations should plan on building value creation programs in such a way that success is likely to occur. When the needs of organizations become broader and more complicated, it never hurts to ask for help from experienced professionals. Time and resources must be available to attempt and sustain advanced Tier 3* projects. In general a team should be composed of these people:

1) Experienced mentors (who have preferably completed multiple projects of various levels of complexity)
2) Mediators (who help organize content experts and contributors when Value Units scales are being used)
3) Data analysts (computer scientists who can tabulate data and create charts efficiently)
4) Program managers or directors (to set time tables, archive successes/failures, help with scheduling, and enforce institutional rigor)

Reports should emphasize the ease of interpretation that comes from using Value Unit scale measures. A Tier 3* Value Analysis (the most complex of logic chains) may look something like this:

Tier 3* Value Measure Analysis - Hip Surgery Bundle Measures - Department of Orthopedic Surgery

Using graphics such as "smiley faces" to point out common cause and special cause variation makes a complicated Tier 3* chart less intimidating and even easier to follow. Colors can also be used to designate if quality or cost elements are creating or sustaining value. Note that a Tier 2 Value Analysis just uses one or more subcomponents for primary value measures with a subcomponent in the other category serving as a balance measure. A Tier 2 chart may look something like this:

Tier 2
Value Measure Analysis
Access to Care and Timely Hospital Discharges

Status	Quality Subcomponents

The two "little q" components can be combined into a Quality component value if desired. Alternatively, a quality and a cost component can both be measured as "balance" measures to make sure that cost does not rise and that a specific quality outcome measure does not suffer. This type of reporting begins to show the significant leap of complexity that takes place when a group begins a Tier 3 project versus a Tier 2 project. Even a Tier 2 analysis chart, such as the one shown here, looks simple but requires significant effort to create the logic behind the Value Unit scales and reliable data collection. As this chapter emphasizes, it is always better to start off with simple projects. A Tier 1 chart would further reduce the report to something like this:

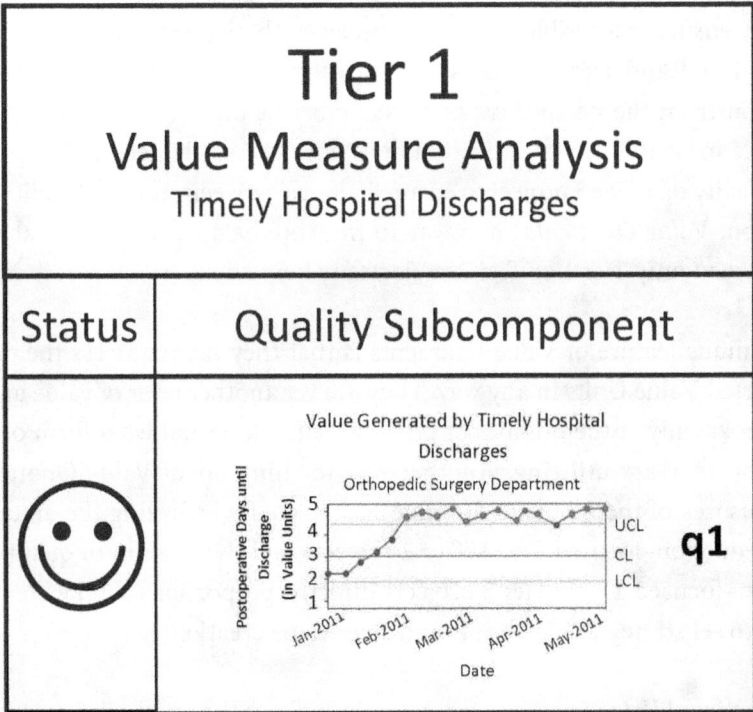

Tier 1
Value Measure Analysis
Timely Hospital Discharges

Status	Quality Subcomponent
🙂	Value Generated by Timely Hospital Discharges Orthopedic Surgery Department *Postoperative Days until Discharge (in Value Units)* 5, 4, 3, 2, 1 Jan-2011, Feb-2011, Mar-2011, Apr-2011, May-2011 UCL, CL, LCL **q1** Date

Use these box-charts to visualize how value creation efforts can follow a step-by-step evolution. Tier 1 analyses can lead to Tier 2 analyses. Three simple Tier 1 projects might be able to be measured together to form a Tier 2 project. Tier 1 and Tier 2 projects might then be combined for form an early Tier 3 project.

When Tier 3 projects grow large enough they will measure total cost of care with quality-outcome balance measures in place to ensure value creation.

Value Quotients

Since most organizations are likely to begin with Tier 1 and Tier 2 value creation projects, another practical concept needs to be presented. First, it must be noted that Tier 3 projects can show multiple cost and quality variables together, ensuring a visible balance between both elements during value creation. Tier 1 and Tier 2 projects, on the other hand, usually only show value creation from the perspective of one side or the other (cost or quality +/- a balance measure). An organization does not necessarily need to jump to the complexity of a Tier 3 project to ensure balance between cost and quality value creation. *Value Quotients* are a way to measure balance and steer value creation when only Tier 1 or Tier 2 projects are being done.

The unique feature of Value Quotients is that they do not assess the data or converted Value Units in any way. They are yet another layer of value analysis that looks only at the number of projects being done and what form of value creation they are utilizing. Another way to think about Value Quotients is as measures of the numbers of Value Formulas. By analyzing the amount of cost reduction–focused Tier 1/Tier 2 projects and the amount of quality promotion–focused Tier 1/Tier 2 projects directly, proportions can be created in order to set strategic value limits and steer value creation.

A *Directional Value Quotient*, for example, looks at the number of quality promotion projects over the number of cost reduction projects. As value creation ideally includes both quality and cost components, this proportion can be used to set *strategic balance thresholds*.

Example of multiple Tier 1 or Tier 2 value creation projects:

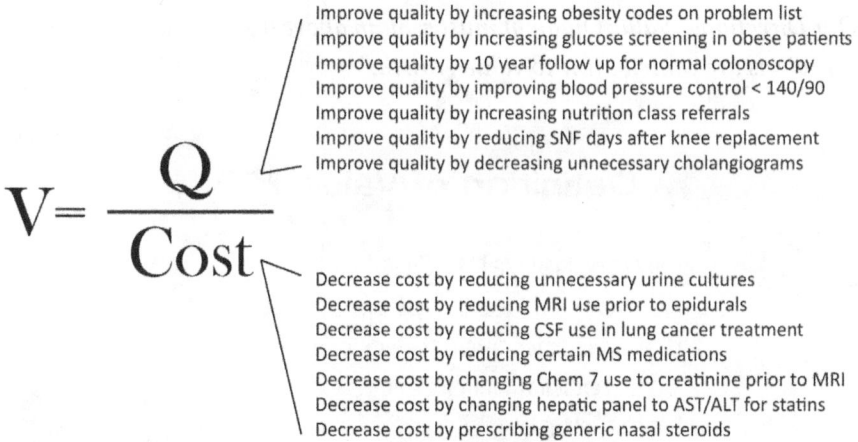

$$V = \frac{Q}{Cost}$$

Improve quality by increasing obesity codes on problem list
Improve quality by increasing glucose screening in obese patients
Improve quality by 10 year follow up for normal colonoscopy
Improve quality by improving blood pressure control < 140/90
Improve quality by increasing nutrition class referrals
Improve quality by reducing SNF days after knee replacement
Improve quality by decreasing unnecessary cholangiograms

Decrease cost by reducing unnecessary urine cultures
Decrease cost by reducing MRI use prior to epidurals
Decrease cost by reducing CSF use in lung cancer treatment
Decrease cost by reducing certain MS medications
Decrease cost by changing Chem 7 use to creatinine prior to MRI
Decrease cost by changing hepatic panel to AST/ALT for statins
Decrease cost by prescribing generic nasal steroids

Calculating a Directional Value Quotient is quite simple. Take, for example, clinical variation reduction (VR) Tier 2 projects at Make Believe Medical Group (MBMG):

Q 20 quality improvement VR standards

$Cost$ 100 cost reduction VR standards

$$\text{Directional Value Quotient} = \frac{20}{100} = 0.2$$

DVQ > 1 means a greater quality focus
DVQ < 1 means a greater cost reduction focus

A Directional Value Quotient of 0.2 (less than 1) shows that there is a significantly greater focus on cost reduction projects. While this is not necessarily bad, the organization may choose to set a *strategic balance threshold* to ensure balance of value creation. A value-statistics professional might say:

"Our Directional Value Quotient must remain above 0.2 to ensure enough quality projects are contributing to value growth."

Definition of Value #20

Directional Value Quotient =
number of quality projects currently
being done over the number of
cost reduction projects currently
being done

A *Growth Value Quotient* is another useful measure that looks at the number of new projects that are underway or being planned. If MBMG, for example, has started 20 quality focused Tier 2 projects and 10 cost reduction Tier 2 projects, then a proportion can be created:

$$\Delta Q \qquad \text{20 quality VR standards started}$$

$$\Delta Cost \qquad \text{10 cost reduction VR standards started}$$

$$\text{Growth Value Quotient} = \frac{20}{10} = 2$$

GVQ > 1 means a greater quality growth
GVQ < 1 means a greater cost reduction growth

A *Growth Value Quotient* of 2 shows that newly started projects are leaning more toward quality creation. A value-statistics professional can now report:

"Our Directional Value Quotient is 0.2 at this time. The Growth Value Quotient of 2 should ensure enough quality projects will contribute to value growth in the future."

Definition of Value #21

Growth Value Quotient = number of quality projects currently being planned or started over the number of cost reduction projects currently being planned or started

The two concepts presented here are simply to illustrate yet another perspective on strategic planning options when it comes to value creation. Simple tracking tools can provide accountability and ensure an organization is heading in the desired direction. Most would agree that it is better to achieve success by design and not by accident.

A Practical Approach to Creating Value Unit Scales

As Value Unit scales can be constructed using many forms of logic and allow for almost infinite flexibility, some practical rules can be used to simplify this important step in value calculations. Following the *Five Golden Steps of Value Unit Scale Creation* can help bring consistency to value creation projects and allow for possible combination of lower-tier projects into Tier 3 projects at a future time.

The Five Golden Steps of Value Unit Scale Creation

Golden Step #1: Chart the Clinical Variation

Pull either quality or cost data on a specific topic in health care that demonstrates variation of practice between providers or parts of an institution and create a chart that illustrates the variance.

The following is an example of cost (charge) data that shows variation between providers:

Average Pre-Clinical-Standard Charges per Patient per Year (US Dollars)

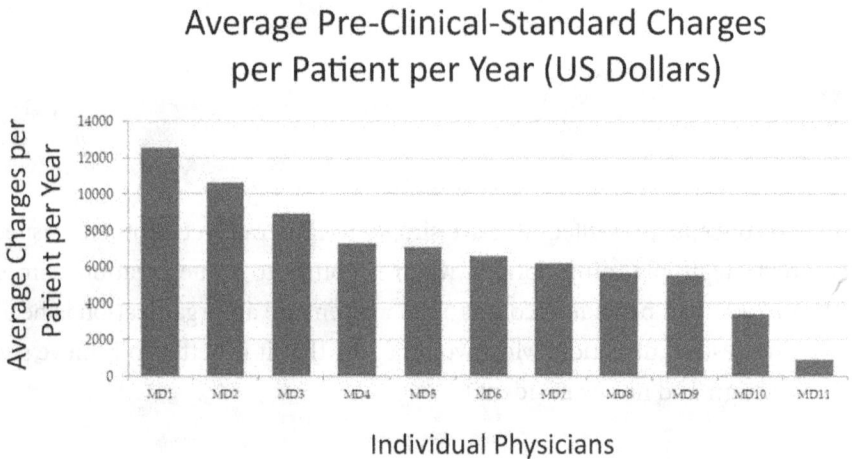

Individual Physicians

In this example we see that it costs $13,000 per patient per year for MD1 (the first doctor) to take care of a patient with a certain medical condition. It takes MD11 (the doctor farthest to the right), on the other hand, only $1,000 per patient per year to take care of patients with the same medical condition. There is a 13-fold variance in the charges.

Golden Step #2: Create the Logic for the Upper Half of the Value Scale

In clinical scenarios a group of local health care providers (and potentially staff and patients) need to decide what would create value to the patient using the logic of *the* Value Equation. In the aforementioned example, a cost reduction project, this group of "content experts" must decide how much savings represents a little value creation and how much clearly represents a significant amount of value creation. As previously mentioned, clinical variation reduction is a methodology for helping groups arrive at this logic. Let us pretend that a group has decided that a cost of more than $10,000/patient/year generates no value for the patient and that a cost of less than $4,000/patient/year generates a lot of value for the patient.

Golden Step #3: Set the Upper Half of the Value Scale

When assigning numbers to the upper part of the Value Unit Scale (i.e., the objective or subjective measures), two practical options are recommended. The first option is to look at the original variation data and assign the highest and lowest numbers to the scale based on the logic created in Golden Step #2. In this case, lowering the cost creates more value, so the $13,000/patient would be on the left side of the scale and the $1,000/patient would be on the right side of the scale. The second option is to utilize the logic created in Golden Step #2 to help shape the scale. The logic tells us that numbers above $10,000/patient generate no value to the patient and that numbers below $4,000/patient generate a lot of value. A value-statistics professional could consider putting $10,000 on the left side of the scale and $4,000 on the right side of the scale.

Golden Step #4: Consider Resetting the Scale to Encourage Value Creation

Although both basic options noted in Golden Step #3 can be used, sometimes a middle ground can also be considered for the purpose of encouraging value creation. As the variation data shows us that two providers have already been able to achieve treatment costs below $4,000, the upper half of the Value Unit scale can "reward" excellent performance by showing numbers at or below $1,000. Accordingly, only two providers' costs were above $10,000/patient, so the scale does not need to show numbers above the $10,000/patient amount as the amount of value generated will be zero anyway.

Therefore, a scale could also be constructed showing $10,000/patient on the left and $1,000/patient toward the right. Recall that the Value Unit half of the scale will always increase from left to right.

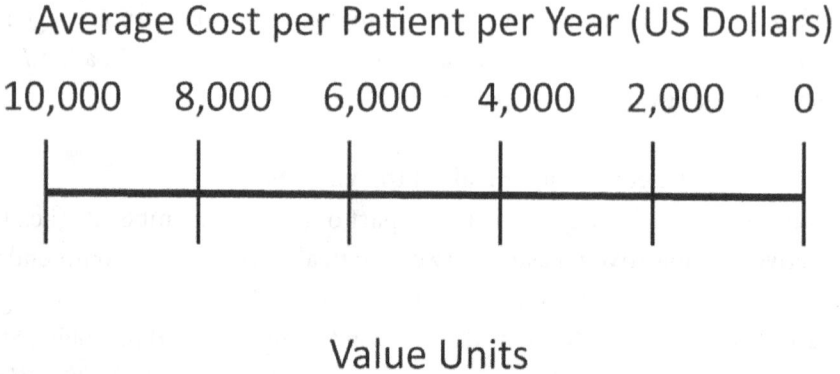

Average Cost per Patient per Year (US Dollars)

10,000   8,000   6,000   4,000   2,000   0

Value Units

Golden Step #5: Complete the Value Unit Scale by Assigning Value Units
Assign a range of Value Units to the lower half of the Value Unit scale from 0 to 5 or 0 to 10—whatever would be more practical for the given scenario—favoring ease of calculations for combining Value Unit run charts and data.

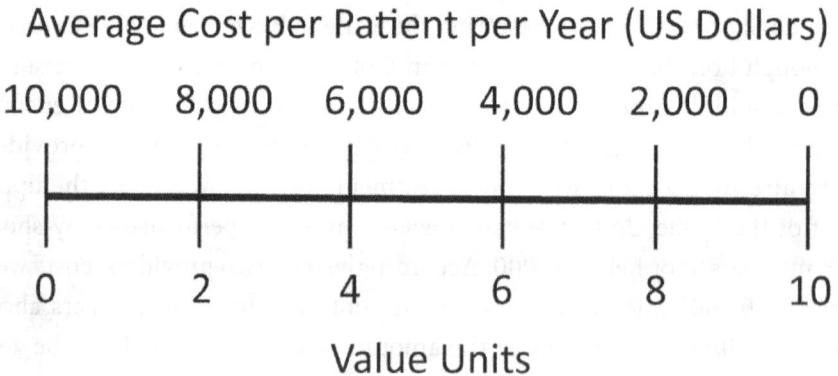

Average Cost per Patient per Year (US Dollars)

10,000   8,000   6,000   4,000   2,000   0

0   2   4   6   8   10

Value Units

Recall that Tier 3 value creation projects will result in combining the Value Units directly and in the form of run charts. As such, the lower half of the Value Unit scale must have consistent logic. Another reasonable consideration is recognizing that providing a service or product for free is not realistic. Therefore, setting the right side of the scale to $1,000 or $500 might be a better choice than allowing it to go down to $0.

Finally, it is very important to emphasize that **Golden Step #5 always recommends starting the Value Unit scale with 0**. While this concept was not illustrated in previous examples, in a practical world it is often advantageous to have a limit where 0 value is generated. It should also be noted here that **negative Value Units are never recommended** due to the unnecessary complexity it adds to calculations.

12

THE IMPORTANCE OF VALUE IN MEDICINE TODAY

"The time is always right to do what is right."—Martin Luther King Jr.

The concept of using value to measure how health systems and providers communicate with their patients and deliver care is growing in popularity. This type of value always means **value to the patient**. Those who counsel about or provide medical services commonly agree with those who receive care that this is the common ground that begins the conversation about value creation.

The word *value* itself is also much more palatable than the sometimes controversial goals of "reducing charges/costs" or "only increasing/maintaining quality." Reducing costs quickly translates to "reducing revenue," which can upset some providers or revenue-cycle professionals. Increasing quality is less visceral but can also strongly induce guilt within a provider group if the goals are not being met. While these individual points and conversations do need to occur, using value terminology is an efficient way to bridge the gap without spooking finance folks or setting practitioners on edge.

Ultimately the goal is the same regardless of terminology or calculation preference. We must all start at our common ground.

Stewardship of the Commons—Why Efforts Such as Value Creation and Clinical Variation Reduction Are Important in Medicine Today

Elinor Ostrom was the first woman awarded the Nobel Prize in economics. She emphasized how humans and ecosystems interact to provide "long-term sustainable resource yields"(*Beyond the tragedy of the commons*, Stockholm Whiteboard Seminars, 2009). She showed how grazing lands, fisheries, forests, and other natural resources have been protected and allocated by humans for thousands of years so as to prevent ecosystem collapse. Put simply, if a community had grazing lands in the middle of several villages, the groups had to learn to share and protect "the commons." If one group allowed their sheep to over-eat the common grazing lands, the other sheep would die and everyone would starve. Focusing on value creation calculations and grassroots efforts such as clinical variation reduction carries on the tradition of the *Stewardship of the Commons*. Rising health care costs are not sustainable. Even worse, rising costs are not even increasing the quality of care being provided. High-quality, affordable health care with good access for all represents a "commons" that is worth retrieving and protecting. With an emphasis on ease of calculations and methodologies focused on improved care and decreased costs, value creation statistics and engagement techniques such as clinical variation reduction employ the most fundamental human quality within health care: the desire to help our neighbors and preserve the gift of sustainable health care for future generations to come.

Parting Words

Whether writing basic Consensus Value surveys or strategically planning the most complicated "mega bundle," the principles of value creation should never be forgotten. Value comes from people. Measuring what people say, what happens to people, or what benefits people in some way ultimately translates to value. Highly complicated value analyses are impressive to behold and generate the most accurate information. For some decisions, however, this level of detail and accuracy is not needed. *Figure out what you can do, how accurate you can be, and then create a practical plan with the resources available.*

Start small but dream large. Master value analysis one bite at a time until the entire whale is consumed.

ABOUT THE AUTHOR

Dr. Veko J. Vahamaki is an internationally experienced physician who practices medicine in the San Francisco Bay Area. He is a national forum speaker on Value at the Group Practice Improvement Network (GPIN) and Institute for Healthcare Improvement (IHI).

It was his professional work in clinical variation reduction that inspired Dr. Vahamaki to improve the function of healthcare systems. His experiences as an advisor for the California Improvement Network (CIN) Action Group to Address Variation of Care and as a Medical Director for Diagnostic Coding at the Palo Alto Medical Foundation, combined with research, led to his book, *Value-Driven Healthcare: A Medical Professional's Guide to Measuring Value and Addressing Total Cost of Care*. Dr. Vahamaki is Adjunct Clinical Faculty at Stanford University School of Medicine. He is married with two sons.

www.ingramcontent.com/pod-product-compliance
Lightning Source LLC
Chambersburg PA
CBHW071133280326
41935CB00010B/1206